Praise for *Paws for the Good Stuff:*

A cat lover's journal for creating a purrfectly pawsitive life!

Carlyn Montes De Oca has created the purr-fect Cat-itude Gratitude journal, not only as a way to celebrate the cats that rule your heart — but to make your own heart sing. *Paws for the Good Stuff* creates twice-daily five-minute empowerment moments, a no-brainer for anyone who wants to feel happier, reduce stress, and model their cat's paw-sitivity. My Karma-Kat gives it all-paws-up!

> — **Amy Shojai,** *CABC, nationally known pet care expert, founder of the Cat Writer's Association, author of more than 35 pet care books*

Paws for the Good Stuff: A Cat Lover's Journal for Creating a Purrfectly Pawsitive Life, is a guided journey toward positivity and joy with your cat as your Sherpa. We all know our cats make our lives better, but this journal captures that feeling to create true change in your approach to life.

> — **Jennifer Steketee,** *DVM, Executive Director, Santa Fe Animal Shelter*

Paws for the Good Stuff is an invitation to open our hearts and allow our feline family members to guide us into a deeper sense of connection with them — and with ourselves. With this unique journal and just five minutes a day, you'll create a practice that brings more mindfulness, more gratitude, and more joy to your life, all day long. Carlyn's sweet and playful prompts will put a smile on your face and help you make happiness and positivity a habit — all with the help of your wise and wonderful cat.

> — **Jan Allegretti,** *D.Vet.Hom., author of "The Complete Holistic Dog Book: Home Health Care for Our Canine Companions"*

Paws for the Good Stuff is a "pawsitvely" unique and creative approach to create a strong bond between you and your cat.

> — **Tim Link,** *Best-selling author of "Talking with Dogs and Cats" and "Wagging Tales"*

Your Kitty Kat knows you better than you do, you just need to stop and listen to their "Meow." Carlyn Montes De Oca showed us this in her first book, *Dog as My Doctor, Cat as my Nurse*. In *Paws for the Good Stuff*, she demonstrates how to take your wellbeing to the next level through the simple and powerful practice of gratitude. If you love cat and want to feel more joy, this is the book for you!

> — **Heidi Selexa,** *Award-winning radio personality, film producer, actress, and comedian*

I've known Carlyn Montes De Oca for many years — and always viewed her as primarily a d-a-w-g person. While she is one of the funniest people I've ever met in my life, I have to take her seriously now because she has finally written an absolutely wonderful book about cats. I am a total cat lover. This journal tugged at my heartstrings. It touches on so many things I value including an infinite love of cats, mindfulness, gratitude, and being in the present moment. *Paws for the Good Stuff*, is a totally feel good book that will help anyone who uses it enjoy their life with their feline(s) more than ever.

> — **Ashley Warrenton Smith,** *CEO Catalyst Coaching and Training, Co-Founder, Dancing with Source*

Whether asleep on your lap, resting by your side, or wide awake on your head wondering when you'll get up to feed them, cats are the furry corrective for the soul. Carlyn Montes De Oca knows this. She also knows how to make the most of one of the happiest companionships you'll ever have. To read *Paws for the Good Stuff* is to practically hear the purr of joy and peace on your chest, even if it is at 4 am.

> — **Francesco Marciuliano,** *Author of "I Could Pee on This and Other Poems by Cats"*

From the award-winning author of
Dog as My Doctor, Cat as My Nurse

Paws for the Good Stuff

A cat lover's journal
for creating a purrfectly pawsitive life!

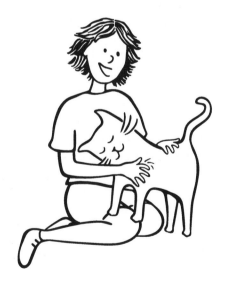

By Carlyn Montes De Oca
Illustrations & Design by Giulia Notari

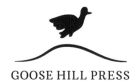

GOOSE HILL PRESS

Paws for the Good Stuff

A cat lover's journal for creating a purrfectly pawsitive life

First Edition Published 2020

Printed in the United States of America

Print ISBN: 978-0-9997812-1-0

Illustration & design by Giulia Notari

For special orders, bulk purchases, sales promotions, corporate sales, fund-raising and more contact Publisher@GooseHillPress.com.

This book is not intended as a substitute for the medical advice of physicians or veterinarians. The reader should regularly consult a physician in matters relating to his or her health and a veterinarian regarding their companion animal's health, particularly with respect to symptoms that may require diagnosis or medical attention.

To all who love and cherish their feline friends....
may your cat help you live your most
pawsitive life.

And to Jester and Cody,
my friends, my inspiration, my soul.
Until we meet again on that rainbow bridge.

This Journal Belongs to

_____

and to

_____

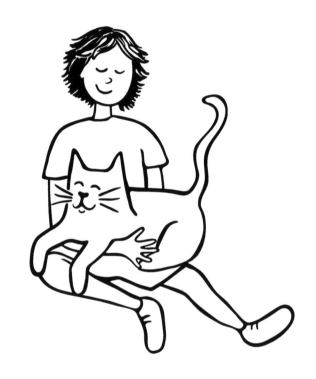

friends forever

Me & My Best Friend

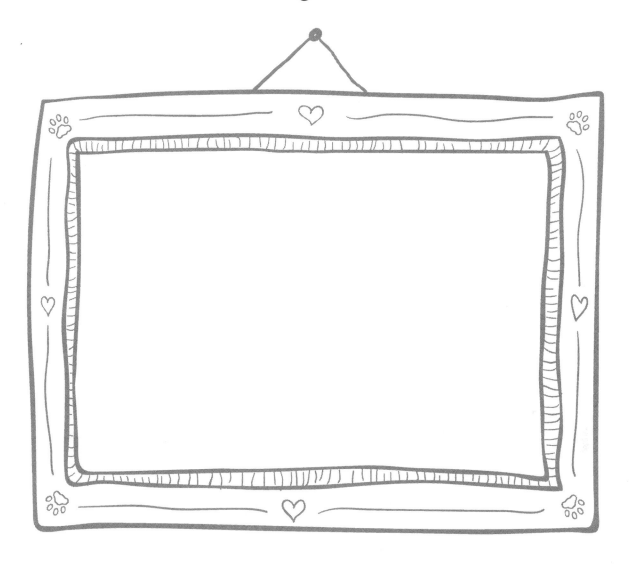

Add a selfie of you with your kitty in the frame above.
If you don't have a photo, then get creative and doodle or draw one.
Have fun! This is your *pawsitive* journal after all.

Purr · fect
Paws · i · tiv · i · ty

an optimistic attitude
inspired by cats

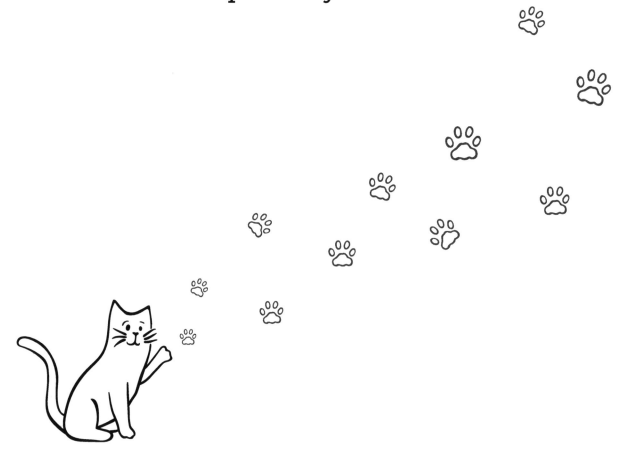

Contents

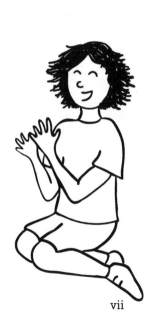

"

I have found it is surprisingly difficult to remain sad when a cat is doing its level best to sandpaper one's cheeks.

R.L. LAFEVERS

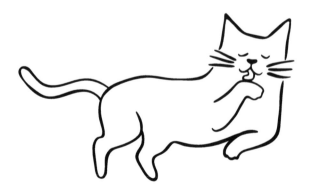

Why Paws for the Good Stuff?

When was the last time you felt *purrfectly pawsitive?*

Were you smiling? Did you feel on top of the world? What did your heart dare to dream?

Having a *pawsitive* outlook helps us see life's challenges differently. When we laugh the world feels brighter. When we smile, others smile with us. When we feel optimistic, our energy is contagious.

We can't be happy 100% of the time and that's OK. Sadness, grief, and anger are natural yet they can feel as painful as a physical injury. Sometimes we need a wounded heart to remind us that we are human and to encourage us to feel compassion towards our fellow earthlings — human and animal.

The problem becomes when we allow our negative feelings to linger, become chronic, and adversely affect our quality of life. Not only do we suffer but those around us feel our negative energy too. When we become captive to this downward spiral, happiness feels forever out of reach.

Gratitude → Pawsitivity → Happiness

I am not naturally optimistic. My smiles come from a choice I made years ago to be happier by choosing a *pawsitive* mindset which I cultivate daily through a variety of practices. One of these habits includes my animal friends. Over the years, surrounded by rescue animals, I've discovered that when I tune into them, open my heart to their timeless wisdom, and express my gratitude for all they are and all they teach me; this is when my attitude shifts for the better.

Our feline BFFS model qualities like playfulness, grace, appreciation, enthusiasm, joy, trust, and unconditional love; *pawsitive* qualities we humans can greatly benefit from. Becoming aware that our animal friends are more than just pets — and are instead nature's delightful teachers, life's wise masters, and sages of simplicity — is when we open the door to the *pawsitive*, to greater happiness, and ultimately to our own transformation.

I created *Paws for the Good Stuff* as a follow-up to my award-winning book, *Dog as My Doctor, Cat as My Nurse,* when I noticed that my clients were missing one life-changing key to their wellness — a gratitude practice. Starting your day with a healthy breakfast is excellent, but for the mind and spirit, gratitude is the breakfast of champions.

I also made this journal for myself because I want to feel happier in my daily life, to nurture my emotional resilience, and to live a life of greater connection with my animal friends — and I'd like others to do the same.

If you love cats and feel their loving pawprints on your heart, I welcome you to join me on this journey of exploration, empowerment, and appreciation. I also encourage you to let others know this unique journal is available. Happier people create a more hopeful world — and boy do we need that now more than ever!

We can use a helping hand from time to time, but for those of us who feel that happiness is where our cat lies, there is nothing better than a loving paw to crack open our hearts and transform our lives. And in transforming ourselves, we take a giant step in changing our world too.

Stay *Pawsitive!*

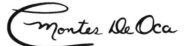

Discoveries & Benefits

The Power of Your Subconscious

Your subconscious mind is most active during two times of the day: when you first wake up in the morning and when you are drifting off to sleep. These highly receptive states are the best moments to give your brain and body time to pause, take note, and discover how your feline BFF can inspire you to feel more *pawsitive*.

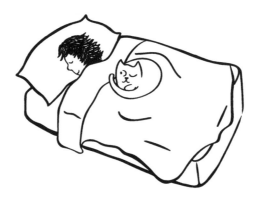

Inside This Journal You Will Discover...

- 🐾 6 months (24 weeks) of journal pages **plus 2 bonus weeks**

- 🐾 Weekly Challenges every 7 days

- 🐾 Monthly Milestones every 28 days

- 🐾 Fun illustrations

- 🐾 Feline fun facts

- 🐾 Daily inspiring quotes

- 🐾 An exclusive link to 6 short videos with helpful tips to deepen your journaling experience

- 🐾 *Get Curious* prompts to enhance, enrich, and enliven your journaling adventure

Discoveries & Benefits

9 Ways *Paws for the Good Stuff* Can Benefit Your Life...

- 🐾 Inspires you to have for a more joyful day

- 🐾 Promotes mental & emotional well-being

- 🐾 Increases mindfulness

- 🐾 Helps replace negative thoughts with a *pawsitive* mindset

- 🐾 Boosts your emotional intelligence

- 🐾 Allows you to connect with your cat in a unique and meaningful way

- 🐾 Helps you enjoy a better night's sleep by reflecting on your *pawsitive* day

- 🐾 Results in a one-of-a-kind keepsake of lasting memories shared with your beloved kitty

- 🐾 Reminds you that **you** are *'the good stuff!'*

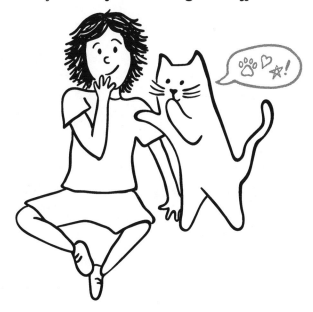

But, But, But, And...

But *I feel resistant.*
And you are not alone. Humans are resistant to change. Yet change is how we grow, discover who we are, and what we are capable of becoming. This journal will help you get out of your head and move into your heart; the number one place our cats like to live.

But *I don't have time.*
And if you don't have 5 minutes to give yourself in the morning and at night, then you are absolutely right — this journal is not for you. If you want to feel happier, more *pawsitive*, and to take your life to the next level, then give yourself a gift of at least 5 minutes of quality time every single day and night.

But *I've done journals before and they haven't worked for me.*
And we've all tried things that haven't worked. But *Paws for the Good Stuff* is a unique journal specifically created for cat lovers. No other journal exists quite like it. What would you lose by trying a new approach based upon your connection, friendship, and love for your feline friend? If you learn one thing about yourself throughout this journey, if you feel even a little bit happier, a tad more *pawsitive* — won't it be worth it?

Pawsitive Tips

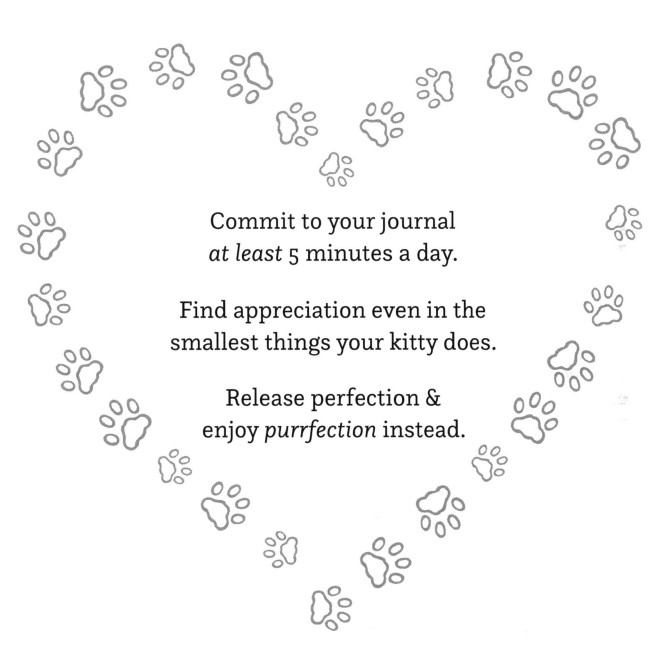

Commit to your journal
at least 5 minutes a day.

Find appreciation even in the
smallest things your kitty does.

Release perfection &
enjoy *purrfection* instead.

How to Use Your Journal

Keep *Paws for the Good Stuff* and your favorite writing instrument on the nightstand next to your bed. In the morning, as soon as you wake up, take a few deep breaths to get yourself ready.

Open your journal and take a few minutes to answer the three short questions in the AM section.

At bedtime answer the questions in the PM section. As you drift off to sleep, do the last prompt in your mind (and your heart) for 1 – 2 minutes before you .....zzzzzzz.

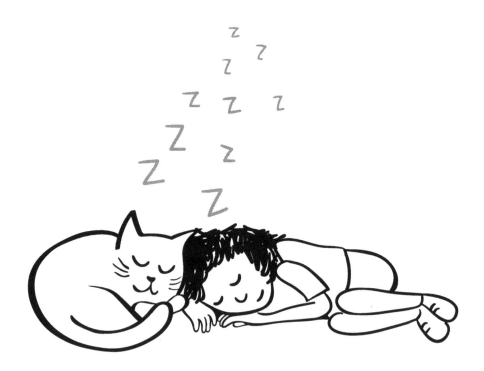

Pawsitive Power Words

Every morning you will be asked to choose one *Pawsitive Power Word* to use throughout your day. Choose any word that makes you feel more empowered, more balanced, and that lifts your spirit. If you have trouble coming up with one on your own, borrow one of ours!

gratitude kindness peaceful delight

inspiring grace empathy

love insight hope forgiveness

friendship fun trust magic

appreciation joy gratitude

playful wisdom transformation

abundance

Sample Page

Your house will always be blessed with love, laughter and friendship if you have a cat.

LEWIS CARROLL

Date   March 1

My Pawsitive Power Word of the Day   Playful

am

This morning I woke up feeling   Glum

As I go through my day I wish to feel   Happier

I am grateful to my cat,   Cody   because I was feeling glum then he jumped on my chest and made me laugh.

How can my kitty BFF inspire me to have a more *pawsitive* day? (If you get stuck, use your power word.)

if I feel glum again, I'm going to remember that playing with Cody makes me feel happy. Then, I'm going to play with him!

pm

3 *pawsitive* things that happened to me today were...

🐾   I was thinking about Cody and smiling when Joe, my co-worker, smiled back at me.

🐾   I got stuck in traffic but instead of getting upset, I sang my favorite songs in the car.

🐾   I took time for myself and Cody to do nothing but lay on the couch and feel his purr on my chest.

Tonight as I drift off to sleep I will send happiness & *pawsitive* thoughts to...

Joe.

Sample Page

Life isn't about finding yourself, life is about creating yourself.

GEORGE BERNARD SHAW

Date   **March 2**

My Pawsitive Power Word of the Day   **Kindness**

am

This morning I woke up feeling   **Hopeful**

As I go through my day I wish to feel   **More connection to people I love.**

I am grateful to my cat,   **Jester**   because   **Regardless of what happens in my day, he makes me feel loved.**

How can my kitty BFF inspire me to have a more *pawsitive* day? (If you get stuck, use your power word.)

I'm going to make a donaton to a local cat rescue. I know how much every little bit counts.

pm

3 *pawsitive* things that happened to me today were...

- **I turned my cell phone off and took a walk at lunchtime.**
- **I talked to a childhood friend of mine on the phone and it was great to connect.**
- **The woman at the cat rescue was so grateful and that made me feel super!**

Tonight as I drift off to sleep I will send happiness & *pawsitive* thoughts to...

The kitties in the rescue, just like my Jester, who are waiting to find for their forever homes.

My Pawsitive Commitment

I, _____
commit to creating a purrfectly *pawsitive* life by
writing in my *Paws for the Good Stuff* journal
every morning and evening.

I commit to embark on my *pawsitive* journey
with an open mind, a little focus, and a sense of fun!

I commit to celebrate every 30 days by reminding
myself how amazing I am. Of course, I will also make sure
to let my cat know that she/he is pretty darn stellar too!

Today's Date

_____

Your Signature

_____

And now...
Paws for the Good Stuff!

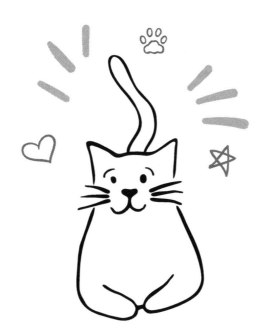

Thousands of years ago, cats were worshiped as gods.
Cats have never forgotten this.

TERRY PRATCHETT

Date _____

My *Pawsitive* Power Word of the Day _____

am

This morning I woke up feeling _____

As I go through my day I wish to feel _____

I am grateful to my cat, _____ because _____

How can my kitty BFF inspire me to have a more *pawsitive* day? (If you get stuck, use your power word.)

_____

pm

3 *pawsitive* things that happened to me today were...

🐾 _____

🐾 _____

🐾 _____

Tonight as I drift off to sleep I will send happiness & *pawsitive* thoughts to...

_____

Fall seven times; stand up eight.

JAPANESE PROVERB

Date _____

My *Pawsitive* Power Word of the Day _____

am

This morning I woke up feeling _____

As I go through my day I wish to feel _____

I am grateful to my cat, _____ because _____

How can my kitty BFF inspire me to have a more *pawsitive* day? (If you get stuck, use your power word.)

_____

pm

3 *pawsitive* things that happened to me today were...

🐾 _____

🐾 _____

🐾 _____

Tonight as I drift off to sleep I will send happiness & *pawsitive* thoughts to...

_____

Purr more, hiss less.

LINDA C. MARCHMAN

Date _____

My *Pawsitive* Power Word of the Day _____

am

This morning I woke up feeling _____

As I go through my day I wish to feel _____

I am grateful to my cat, _____ because _____

How can my kitty BFF inspire me to have a more *pawsitive* day? (If you get stuck, use your power word.)

pm

3 *pawsitive* things that happened to me today were...

🐾 _____

🐾 _____

🐾 _____

Tonight as I drift off to sleep I will send happiness & *pawsitive* thoughts to...

Have a mind that's open to everything and attached to nothing.

WAYNE DYER

Date _____

My *Pawsitive* Power Word of the Day _____

am

This morning I woke up feeling _____

As I go through my day I wish to feel _____

I am grateful to my cat, _____ because _____

How can my kitty BFF inspire me to have a more *pawsitive* day? (If you get stuck, use your power word.)

_____

pm

3 *pawsitive* things that happened to me today were...

🐾 _____

🐾 _____

🐾 _____

Tonight as I drift off to sleep I will send happiness & *pawsitive* thoughts to...

_____

Way down deep, we're all motivated by the same urges.
Cats have the courage to live by them.

JIM DAVIS

Date _____

My *Pawsitive* Power Word of the Day _____

am

This morning I woke up feeling _____

As I go through my day I wish to feel _____

I am grateful to my cat, _____ because _____

How can my kitty BFF inspire me to have a more *pawsitive* day? (If you get stuck, use your power word.)

_____

pm

3 *pawsitive* things that happened to me today were...

🐾 _____

🐾 _____

🐾 _____

Tonight as I drift off to sleep I will send happiness & *pawsitive* thoughts to...

_____

A bird does not sing because it has an answer.
It sings because it has a song.

CHINESE PROVERB

Date _____

My *Pawsitive* Power Word of the Day _____

am

This morning I woke up feeling _____

As I go through my day I wish to feel _____

I am grateful to my cat, _____ because _____

How can my kitty BFF inspire me to have a more *pawsitive* day? (If you get stuck, use your power word.)

pm

3 *pawsitive* things that happened to me today were...

🐾 _____

🐾 _____

🐾 _____

Tonight as I drift off to sleep I will send happiness & *pawsitive* thoughts to...

The cat has too much spirit to have no heart.

ERNEST MENAUL

The Seventh Day Challenge

How did you and your cat first meet?
What drew you to each other?

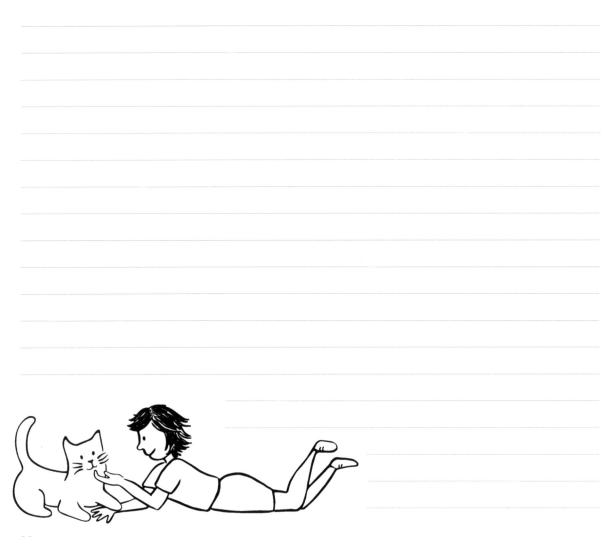

When you let your own light shine, you unconsciously
give others permission to do the same.

NELSON MANDELA

Date _____

My *Pawsitive* Power Word of the Day _____

am

This morning I woke up feeling _____

As I go through my day I wish to feel _____

I am grateful to my cat, _____ because _____

How can my kitty BFF inspire me to have a more *pawsitive* day? (If you get stuck, use your power word.)

_____

pm

3 *pawsitive* things that happened to me today were...

- 🐾 _____
- 🐾 _____
- 🐾 _____

Tonight as I drift off to sleep I will send happiness & *pawsitive* thoughts to...

_____

There are few things in life more heartwarming
than to be welcomed by a cat.

TAY HOHOFF

Date _____

My *Pawsitive* Power Word of the Day _____

am

This morning I woke up feeling _____

As I go through my day I wish to feel _____

I am grateful to my cat, _____ because _____

How can my kitty BFF inspire me to have a more *pawsitive* day? (If you get stuck, use your power word.)

_____

pm

3 *pawsitive* things that happened to me today were...

🐾 _____

🐾 _____

🐾 _____

Tonight as I drift off to sleep I will send happiness & *pawsitive* thoughts to...

_____

The way to my heart is covered with paw prints.

BARBARA L. DIAMOND

Date _____

My *Pawsitive* Power Word of the Day _____

am

This morning I woke up feeling _____

As I go through my day I wish to feel _____

I am grateful to my cat, _____ because _____

How can my kitty BFF inspire me to have a more *pawsitive* day? (If you get stuck, use your power word.)

_____

pm

3 *pawsitive* things that happened to me today were...

🐾 _____

🐾 _____

🐾 _____

Tonight as I drift off to sleep I will send happiness & *pawsitive* thoughts to...

_____

I've met many thinkers and many cats,
but the wisdom of cats is infinitely superior.

Date _____

My *Pawsitive* Power Word of the Day _____

am

This morning I woke up feeling _____

As I go through my day I wish to feel _____

I am grateful to my cat, _____ because _____

How can my kitty BFF inspire me to have a more *pawsitive* day? (If you get stuck, use your power word.)

_____

pm

3 *pawsitive* things that happened to me today were...

🐾 _____

🐾 _____

🐾 _____

Tonight as I drift off to sleep I will send happiness & *pawsitive* thoughts to...

_____

Happiness cannot be traveled to, owned, earned, worn or consumed.
Happiness is the spiritual experience of living every minute
with love, grace, and gratitude.

DENIS WAITLEY

Date _____

My *Pawsitive* Power Word of the Day _____

am

This morning I woke up feeling _____

As I go through my day I wish to feel _____

I am grateful to my cat, _____ because _____

How can my kitty BFF inspire me to have a more *pawsitive* day? (If you get stuck, use your power word.)

_____

pm

3 *pawsitive* things that happened to me today were...

🐾 _____

🐾 _____

🐾 _____

Tonight as I drift off to sleep I will send happiness & *pawsitive* thoughts to...

_____

Women and cats will do as they please,
and men and dogs should relax and get used to the idea.

ROBERT A. HEINLEIN

Date _____

My *Pawsitive* Power Word of the Day _____

am

This morning I woke up feeling _____

As I go through my day I wish to feel _____

I am grateful to my cat, _____ because _____

How can my kitty BFF inspire me to have a more *pawsitive* day? (If you get stuck, use your power word.)

pm

3 *pawsitive* things that happened to me today were...

🐾 _____

🐾 _____

🐾 _____

Tonight as I drift off to sleep I will send happiness & *pawsitive* thoughts to...

If opportunity doesn't knock, build a door.
MILTON BERLE

The Seventh Day Challenge

If my cat could talk,
what do I think she/he would want me to know?

That was Zen, this is meow.

AUTHOR UNKNOWN

Date _____

My *Pawsitive* Power Word of the Day _____

am

This morning I woke up feeling _____

As I go through my day I wish to feel _____

I am grateful to my cat, _____ because _____

How can my kitty BFF inspire me to have a more *pawsitive* day? (If you get stuck, use your power word.)

pm

3 *pawsitive* things that happened to me today were...

🐾 _____

🐾 _____

🐾 _____

Tonight as I drift off to sleep I will send happiness & *pawsitive* thoughts to...

No medicine cures what happiness cannot.
GABRIEL GARCÍA MÁRQUEZ

Date _____

My *Pawsitive* Power Word of the Day _____

am

This morning I woke up feeling _____

As I go through my day I wish to feel _____

I am grateful to my cat, _____ because _____

How can my kitty BFF inspire me to have a more *pawsitive* day? (If you get stuck, use your power word.)

_____

pm

3 *pawsitive* things that happened to me today were...

🐾 _____

🐾 _____

🐾 _____

Tonight as I drift off to sleep I will send happiness & *pawsitive* thoughts to...

_____

Cats tell me without effort all that there is to know.

CHARLES BUKOWSKI

Date _____

My *Pawsitive* Power Word of the Day _____

am

This morning I woke up feeling _____

As I go through my day I wish to feel _____

I am grateful to my cat, _____ because _____

How can my kitty BFF inspire me to have a more *pawsitive* day? (If you get stuck, use your power word.)

pm

3 *pawsitive* things that happened to me today were...

🐾 _____

🐾 _____

🐾 _____

Tonight as I drift off to sleep I will send happiness & *pawsitive* thoughts to...

*Since you get more joy out of giving joy to others, you should put
a good deal of thought into the happiness that you are able to give.*

ELEANOR ROOSEVELT

Date _____

My *Pawsitive* Power Word of the Day _____

am

This morning I woke up feeling _____

As I go through my day I wish to feel _____

I am grateful to my cat, _____ because _____

How can my kitty BFF inspire me to have a more *pawsitive* day? (If you get stuck, use your power word.)

_____

pm

3 *pawsitive* things that happened to me today were...

🐾 _____

🐾 _____

🐾 _____

Tonight as I drift off to sleep I will send happiness & *pawsitive* thoughts to...

_____

A meow massages the heart.

STUART MCMILLAN

Date _____

My *Pawsitive* Power Word of the Day _____

am

This morning I woke up feeling _____

As I go through my day I wish to feel _____

I am grateful to my cat, _____ because _____

How can my kitty BFF inspire me to have a more *pawsitive* day? (If you get stuck, use your power word.)

pm

3 *pawsitive* things that happened to me today were...

🐾 _____

🐾 _____

🐾 _____

Tonight as I drift off to sleep I will send happiness & *pawsitive* thoughts to...

There is more to life than increasing its speed.

MAHATMA GANDHI

Date _____

My *Pawsitive* Power Word of the Day _____

am

This morning I woke up feeling _____

As I go through my day I wish to feel _____

I am grateful to my cat, _____ because _____

How can my kitty BFF inspire me to have a more *pawsitive* day? (If you get stuck, use your power word.)

_____

pm

3 *pawsitive* things that happened to me today were...

🐾 _____

🐾 _____

🐾 _____

Tonight as I drift off to sleep I will send happiness & *pawsitive* thoughts to...

_____

No heaven will not ever be Heaven be;
unless my cats are there to welcome me.

AUTHOR UNKNOWN

The Seventh Day Challenge

List 5 *pawsitive* words that best describe your cat.
List 5 *pawsitive* words that best describe you.

1 _____   1 _____

2 _____   2 _____

3 _____   3 _____

4 _____   4 _____

5 _____   5 _____

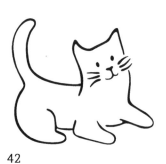

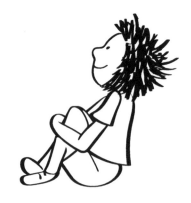

Friendship isn't about whom you have known the longest...
it's about who came and never left your side.
MIKAELA TIU

Did you know?

Our sight is better *and worse* than yours.

Humans see the world in vibrant colors yet we cats possess the ability to see in the dark. But we aren't color blind — we see shades of blue and green. So remember to choose these colors when you buy us toys.

Note: If we look into your eyes and slowly blink, it means we trust you.

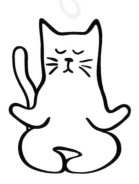

A cat is more intelligent than people believe,
and can be taught any crime.

RALPH WALDO EMERSON

Date _____

My *Pawsitive* Power Word of the Day _____

am

This morning I woke up feeling _____

As I go through my day I wish to feel _____

I am grateful to my cat, _____ because _____

How can my kitty BFF inspire me to have a more *pawsitive* day? (If you get stuck, use your power word.)

pm

3 *pawsitive* things that happened to me today were...

🐾 _____

🐾 _____

🐾 _____

Tonight as I drift off to sleep I will send happiness & *pawsitive* thoughts to...

I am not bound to win, I am bound to be true. I am not bound to succeed,
but I am bound to live up to the light I have.

ABRAHAM LINCOLN

Date _____

My *Pawsitive* Power Word of the Day _____

am

This morning I woke up feeling _____

As I go through my day I wish to feel _____

I am grateful to my cat, _____ because _____

How can my kitty BFF inspire me to have a more *pawsitive* day? (If you get stuck, use your power word.)

pm

3 *pawsitive* things that happened to me today were...

🐾 _____

🐾 _____

🐾 _____

Tonight as I drift off to sleep I will send happiness & *pawsitive* thoughts to...

*A cat has absolute emotional honesty: human beings, for one reason
or another, may hide their feelings, but a cat does not.*

EARNEST HEMINGWAY

Date _____

My *Pawsitive* Power Word of the Day _____

am

This morning I woke up feeling _____

As I go through my day I wish to feel _____

I am grateful to my cat, _____ because _____

How can my kitty BFF inspire me to have a more *pawsitive* day? (If you get stuck, use your power word.)

pm

3 *pawsitive* things that happened to me today were...

🐾 _____

🐾 _____

🐾 _____

Tonight as I drift off to sleep I will send happiness & *pawsitive* thoughts to...

There are those who give with joy, and that joy is their reward.

KHALIL GIBRAN

Date _____

My *Pawsitive* Power Word of the Day _____

am

This morning I woke up feeling _____

As I go through my day I wish to feel _____

I am grateful to my cat, _____ because _____

How can my kitty BFF inspire me to have a more *pawsitive* day? (If you get stuck, use your power word.)

_____

pm

3 *pawsitive* things that happened to me today were...

🐾 _____

🐾 _____

🐾 _____

Tonight as I drift off to sleep I will send happiness & *pawsitive* thoughts to...

_____

If there were to be a universal sound depicting peace,
I would surely vote for the purr.

BARBARA L. DIAMOND

Date _____

My *Pawsitive* Power Word of the Day _____

am

This morning I woke up feeling _____

As I go through my day I wish to feel _____

I am grateful to my cat, _____ because _____

How can my kitty BFF inspire me to have a more *pawsitive* day? (If you get stuck, use your power word.)

_____

pm

3 *pawsitive* things that happened to me today were...

🐾 _____

🐾 _____

🐾 _____

Tonight as I drift off to sleep I will send happiness & *pawsitive* thoughts to...

_____

Shine like the whole universe is yours.

RUMI

Date _____

My *Pawsitive* Power Word of the Day _____

am

This morning I woke up feeling _____

As I go through my day I wish to feel_____

I am grateful to my cat, _____ because _____

How can my kitty BFF inspire me to have a more *pawsitive* day? (If you get stuck, use your power word.)

_____

pm

3 *pawsitive* things that happened to me today were...

🐾 _____

🐾 _____

🐾 _____

Tonight as I drift off to sleep I will send happiness & *pawsitive* thoughts to...

_____

The Pawsitive Monthly Milestone

Create a Memory!

Take a selfie of you and your kitty BFF in your favorite spot together. Send it as a text to someone you appreciate. Or turn it into a fun card and snail mail it to a friend who can use a smile right now.

Place your selfie below.

#PawsForTheGoodStuff 🐾 Spread the *Pawsitivity*!

Share your picture with your online community and use #PawsForTheGoodStuff. Together we can change the world, one *pawsitive* moment at a time.

Get Curious!

Keep it Fresh!

You are in a groove, journaling every morning and evening and discovering new and exciting ways to feel grateful and more *pawsitive*. You are starting to embrace the power in the practice. But if you are also beginning to feel that things are getting a bit repetitive - then it's time to get specific.

LEARN MORE ON HOW TO KEEP IT FRESH AT

PawsForTheGoodStuff.com/GetCurious

Watch my exclusive short video and discover how you can take your journaling experience to the next level.

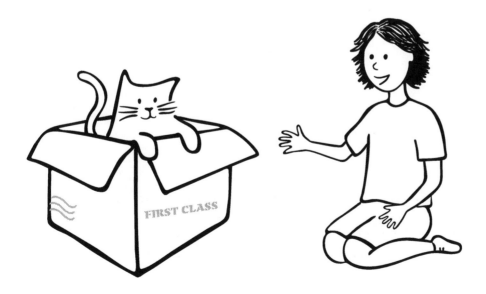

The smallest feline is a masterpiece.

LEONARD DA VINCI

Date _____

My *Pawsitive* Power Word of the Day _____

am

This morning I woke up feeling _____

As I go through my day I wish to feel _____

I am grateful to my cat, _____ because _____

How can my kitty BFF inspire me to have a more *pawsitive* day? (If you get stuck, use your power word.)

pm

3 *pawsitive* things that happened to me today were...

🐾 _____

🐾 _____

🐾 _____

Tonight as I drift off to sleep I will send happiness & *pawsitive* thoughts to...

There is no such thing as a problem without a gift for you in its hands.
You seek problems because you need their gifts.

RICHARD BACH

Date _____

My *Pawsitive* Power Word of the Day _____

am

This morning I woke up feeling _____

As I go through my day I wish to feel _____

I am grateful to my cat, _____ because _____

How can my kitty BFF inspire me to have a more *pawsitive* day? (If you get stuck, use your power word.)

_____

pm

3 *pawsitive* things that happened to me today were...

🐾 _____

🐾 _____

🐾 _____

Tonight as I drift off to sleep I will send happiness & *pawsitive* thoughts to...

_____

Happy is the home with at least one cat.

ITALIAN PROVERB

Date _____

My *Pawsitive* Power Word of the Day _____

am

This morning I woke up feeling _____

As I go through my day I wish to feel _____

I am grateful to my cat, _____ because _____

How can my kitty BFF inspire me to have a more *pawsitive* day? (If you get stuck, use your power word.)

_____

pm

3 *pawsitive* things that happened to me today were...

🐾 _____

🐾 _____

🐾 _____

Tonight as I drift off to sleep I will send happiness & *pawsitive* thoughts to...

_____

I found your paw when I needed a hand for a support.

GAIL CARRIGER

Date _____

My *Pawsitive* Power Word of the Day _____

am

This morning I woke up feeling _____

As I go through my day I wish to feel _____

I am grateful to my cat, _____ because _____

How can my kitty BFF inspire me to have a more *pawsitive* day? (If you get stuck, use your power word.)

_____

pm

3 *pawsitive* things that happened to me today were...

🐾 _____

🐾 _____

🐾 _____

Tonight as I drift off to sleep I will send happiness & *pawsitive* thoughts to...

_____

If purring could be encapsulated, it would be the
most powerful antidepressant on the market.

TERRI GUILLEMETS

Date _____

My *Pawsitive* Power Word of the Day _____

am

This morning I woke up feeling _____

As I go through my day I wish to feel _____

I am grateful to my cat, _____ because _____

How can my kitty BFF inspire me to have a more *pawsitive* day? (If you get stuck, use your power word.)

_____

pm

3 *pawsitive* things that happened to me today were...

🐾 _____

🐾 _____

🐾 _____

Tonight as I drift off to sleep I will send happiness & *pawsitive* thoughts to...

_____

The most wasted of all days is one without laughter.

E.E. CUMMINGS

Date _____

My *Pawsitive* Power Word of the Day _____

am

This morning I woke up feeling _____

As I go through my day I wish to feel _____

I am grateful to my cat, _____ because _____

How can my kitty BFF inspire me to have a more *pawsitive* day? (If you get stuck, use your power word.)

_____

pm

3 *pawsitive* things that happened to me today were...

🐾 _____

🐾 _____

🐾 _____

Tonight as I drift off to sleep I will send happiness & *pawsitive* thoughts to...

_____

What greater gift than the love of a cat?
CHARLES DICKENS

The Seventh Day Challenge

Every day my cat makes me happy.
What can I do to bring more joy to my BFF today?

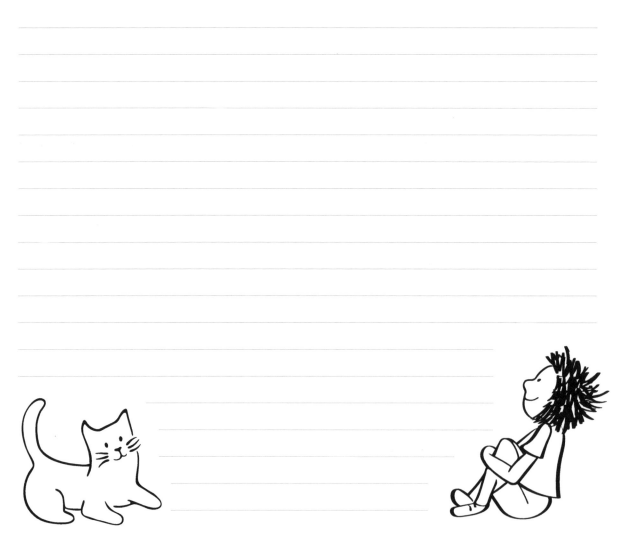

I'd rather have a moment of wonderful than a lifetime of nothing special.

FROM THE MOVIE — STEEL MAGNOLIAS

Date _____

My *Pawsitive* Power Word of the Day _____

am

This morning I woke up feeling _____

As I go through my day I wish to feel _____

I am grateful to my cat, _____ because _____

How can my kitty BFF inspire me to have a more *pawsitive* day? (If you get stuck, use your power word.)

pm

3 *pawsitive* things that happened to me today were...

🐾 _____

🐾 _____

🐾 _____

Tonight as I drift off to sleep I will send happiness & *pawsitive* thoughts to...

I take care of my flowers and my cats. And enjoy food. And that's living.
URSULA ANDRESS

Date _____

My *Pawsitive* Power Word of the Day _____

am

This morning I woke up feeling _____

As I go through my day I wish to feel _____

I am grateful to my cat, _____ because _____

How can my kitty BFF inspire me to have a more *pawsitive* day? (If you get stuck, use your power word.)

pm

3 *pawsitive* things that happened to me today were...

🐾 _____

🐾 _____

🐾 _____

Tonight as I drift off to sleep I will send happiness & *pawsitive* thoughts to...

In our lives, change is unavoidable, loss is unavoidable. In the adaptability and ease with which we experience change, lies our happiness and freedom.

GAUTAMA BUDDHA

Date _____

My *Pawsitive* Power Word of the Day _____

am

This morning I woke up feeling _____

As I go through my day I wish to feel _____

I am grateful to my cat, _____ because _____

How can my kitty BFF inspire me to have a more *pawsitive* day? (If you get stuck, use your power word.)

_____

pm

3 *pawsitive* things that happened to me today were...

🐾 _____

🐾 _____

🐾 _____

Tonight as I drift off to sleep I will send happiness & *pawsitive* thoughts to...

_____

Why do cats sleep so much? Perhaps they've been trusted with some major cosmic task,
an essential law of physics — such as: if there are less than 5 million cats sleeping
at any one time the world will stop spinning. So that when you look at them and think,
'What a lazy, good-for-nothing animal,' they are, in fact, working very, very hard.

KATE ATKINSON

Date _____

My *Pawsitive* Power Word of the Day _____

am

This morning I woke up feeling _____

As I go through my day I wish to feel _____

I am grateful to my cat, _____ because _____

How can my kitty BFF inspire me to have a more *pawsitive* day? (If you get stuck, use your power word.)

pm

3 *pawsitive* things that happened to me today were...

🐾 _____

🐾 _____

🐾 _____

Tonight as I drift off to sleep I will send happiness & *pawsitive* thoughts to...

Cheerfulness is the very flower of health.

PROVERB

Date _____

My *Pawsitive* Power Word of the Day _____

am

This morning I woke up feeling _____

As I go through my day I wish to feel _____

I am grateful to my cat, _____ because _____

How can my kitty BFF inspire me to have a more *pawsitive* day? (If you get stuck, use your power word.)

_____

pm

3 *pawsitive* things that happened to me today were...

🐾 _____

🐾 _____

🐾 _____

Tonight as I drift off to sleep I will send happiness & *pawsitive* thoughts to...

_____

I love cats because I enjoy my home;
and little by little, they become its visible soul.

JEAN COCTEAU

Date _____

My *Pawsitive* Power Word of the Day _____

am

This morning I woke up feeling _____

As I go through my day I wish to feel _____

I am grateful to my cat, _____ because _____

How can my kitty BFF inspire me to have a more *pawsitive* day? (If you get stuck, use your power word.)

_____

pm

3 *pawsitive* things that happened to me today were...

🐾 _____

🐾 _____

🐾 _____

Tonight as I drift off to sleep I will send happiness & *pawsitive* thoughts to...

_____

Love the moment and the energy of that moment
will spread beyond all boundaries.

CORITA KENT

The Seventh Day Challenge

List 7 ways that your cat made you happy this week.

1 _____

2 _____

3 _____

4 _____

5 _____

6 _____

7 _____

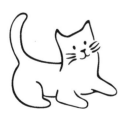

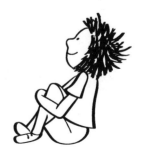

They purr, they pounce, they swat at you when you aren't looking —
cats show their love in unexpected, unexplainable, and downright wonderful ways.

CARLYN MONTES DE OCA

Did you know?

Our noses are like your fingerprints.

Both have unique patterns of ridges and creases. Just as no human fingerprint is the same, no two cats have the same nose print.

Oh and by the way — our sense of smell is 14 times stronger than yours!

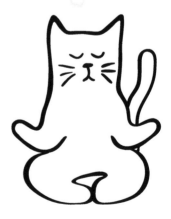

Oh yes, the past can hurt. But you can either run from it, or learn from it.

FROM THE MOVIE — THE LION KING

Date _____

My *Pawsitive* Power Word of the Day _____

am

This morning I woke up feeling _____

As I go through my day I wish to feel _____

I am grateful to my cat, _____ because _____

How can my kitty BFF inspire me to have a more *pawsitive* day? (If you get stuck, use your power word.)

_____

pm

3 *pawsitive* things that happened to me today were...

🐾 _____

🐾 _____

🐾 _____

Tonight as I drift off to sleep I will send happiness & *pawsitive* thoughts to...

_____

The ideal of calm exists in a sitting cat.

JULES REYNARD

Date _____

My *Pawsitive* Power Word of the Day _____

am

This morning I woke up feeling _____

As I go through my day I wish to feel _____

I am grateful to my cat, _____ because _____

How can my kitty BFF inspire me to have a more *pawsitive* day? (If you get stuck, use your power word.)

pm

3 *pawsitive* things that happened to me today were...

🐾 _____

🐾 _____

🐾 _____

Tonight as I drift off to sleep I will send happiness & *pawsitive* thoughts to...

Life is a journey, and if you fall in love with the journey, you will be in love forever.

PETER HAGERTY

Date _____

My *Pawsitive* Power Word of the Day _____

am

This morning I woke up feeling _____

As I go through my day I wish to feel_____

I am grateful to my cat, _____ because _____

How can my kitty BFF inspire me to have a more *pawsitive* day? (If you get stuck, use your power word.)

_____

pm

3 *pawsitive* things that happened to me today were...

🐾 _____

🐾 _____

🐾 _____

Tonight as I drift off to sleep I will send happiness & *pawsitive* thoughts to...

_____

Time spent with cats is never wasted .

SIGMUND FREUD

Date _____

My *Pawsitive* Power Word of the Day _____

am

This morning I woke up feeling _____

As I go through my day I wish to feel _____

I am grateful to my cat, _____ because _____

How can my kitty BFF inspire me to have a more *pawsitive* day? (If you get stuck, use your power word.)

_____

pm

3 *pawsitive* things that happened to me today were...

🐾 _____

🐾 _____

🐾 _____

Tonight as I drift off to sleep I will send happiness & *pawsitive* thoughts to...

_____

People are as happy as they choose to be.

HENRY FORD

Date _____

My *Pawsitive* Power Word of the Day _____

am

This morning I woke up feeling _____

As I go through my day I wish to feel _____

I am grateful to my cat, _____ because _____

How can my kitty BFF inspire me to have a more *pawsitive* day? (If you get stuck, use your power word.)

_____

pm

3 *pawsitive* things that happened to me today were...

🐾 _____

🐾 _____

🐾 _____

Tonight as I drift off to sleep I will send happiness & *pawsitive* thoughts to...

_____

As anyone who has ever been around a cat for any length of time well knows cats have enormous patience with the limitations of the human kind.

CLEVELAND AMORY

Date _____

My *Pawsitive* Power Word of the Day _____

am

This morning I woke up feeling _____

As I go through my day I wish to feel _____

I am grateful to my cat, _____ because _____

How can my kitty BFF inspire me to have a more *pawsitive* day? (If you get stuck, use your power word.)

pm

3 *pawsitive* things that happened to me today were...

🐾 _____

🐾 _____

🐾 _____

Tonight as I drift off to sleep I will send happiness & *pawsitive* thoughts to...

You're going to go through tough times — that's life. But I say,
'Nothing happens to you, it happens for you.' See the positive in negative events.

JOEL OSTEEN

The Seventh Day Challenge

If you love cats, then you probably LOVE their purr.
When your cat purrs, what do you feel he/she is trying to tell you?

It is impossible to keep a straight face in the presence of one or more kittens.

CYNTHIA E. VARNADO

Date _____

My *Pawsitive* Power Word of the Day _____

am

This morning I woke up feeling _____

As I go through my day I wish to feel _____

I am grateful to my cat, _____ because _____

How can my kitty BFF inspire me to have a more *pawsitive* day? (If you get stuck, use your power word.)

_____

pm

3 *pawsitive* things that happened to me today were...

🐾 _____

🐾 _____

🐾 _____

Tonight as I drift off to sleep I will send happiness & *pawsitive* thoughts to...

_____

A good laugh is sunshine in the house.

WILLIAM MAKEPEACE THACKERAY

Date _____

My *Pawsitive* Power Word of the Day _____

am

This morning I woke up feeling _____

As I go through my day I wish to feel _____

I am grateful to my cat, _____ because _____

How can my kitty BFF inspire me to have a more *pawsitive* day? (If you get stuck, use your power word.)

_____

pm

3 *pawsitive* things that happened to me today were...

🐾 _____

🐾 _____

🐾 _____

Tonight as I drift off to sleep I will send happiness & *pawsitive* thoughts to...

_____

All you need is love and a cat.

AUTHOR UNKNOWN

Date _____

My *Pawsitive* Power Word of the Day _____

am

This morning I woke up feeling _____

As I go through my day I wish to feel _____

I am grateful to my cat, _____ because _____

How can my kitty BFF inspire me to have a more *pawsitive* day? (If you get stuck, use your power word.)

pm

3 *pawsitive* things that happened to me today were...

🐾 _____

🐾 _____

🐾 _____

Tonight as I drift off to sleep I will send happiness & *pawsitive* thoughts to...

The butterfly counts not months but moments, and has time enough.

RABINDRANATH TAGORE

Date _____

My *Pawsitive* Power Word of the Day _____

am

This morning I woke up feeling _____

As I go through my day I wish to feel _____

I am grateful to my cat, _____ because _____

How can my kitty BFF inspire me to have a more *pawsitive* day? (If you get stuck, use your power word.)

_____

pm

3 *pawsitive* things that happened to me today were...

🐾 _____

🐾 _____

🐾 _____

Tonight as I drift off to sleep I will send happiness & *pawsitive* thoughts to...

_____

Cats seem to go on the principle that it never does any harm to ask for what you want.

JOSEPH WOOD KRUTCH

Date _____

My *Pawsitive* Power Word of the Day _____

am

This morning I woke up feeling _____

As I go through my day I wish to feel _____

I am grateful to my cat, _____ because _____

How can my kitty BFF inspire me to have a more *pawsitive* day? (If you get stuck, use your power word.)

pm

3 *pawsitive* things that happened to me today were...

🐾 _____

🐾 _____

🐾 _____

Tonight as I drift off to sleep I will send happiness & *pawsitive* thoughts to...

Believe it is possible and take a step. Then tomorrow take another one
and the day after that another. In a year, you'll have climbed at least one mountain.

CARLYN MONTES DE OCA

Date _____

My *Pawsitive* Power Word of the Day _____

am

This morning I woke up feeling _____

As I go through my day I wish to feel _____

I am grateful to my cat, _____ because _____

How can my kitty BFF inspire me to have a more *pawsitive* day? (If you get stuck, use your power word.)

pm

3 *pawsitive* things that happened to me today were...

🐾 _____

🐾 _____

🐾 _____

Tonight as I drift off to sleep I will send happiness & *pawsitive* thoughts to...

The Pawsitive Monthly Milestone

Create a Kitty Treasure Hunt!

Hide a catnip toy in an empty box, leave a yummy treat near a scratching post, or leave a ping pong ball in your bathtub. Then sit back and enjoy watching your cat discover, uncover, and recover from all the fun!

Take pictures and place one or more below.

#PawsForTheGoodStuff 🐾 Spread the *Pawsitivity*!

Share your picture with your online community and use #PawsForTheGoodStuff. Together we can change the world, one *pawsitive* moment at a time.

Get Curious!

Use Your Senses!

Last month you learned how to get more specific as you journal.
When we get specific, magic begins to happen in our daily life.
How about creating more magic? You can do this by waking up
to the world of your 5 senses.

LEARN MORE ON HOW TO USE YOUR SENSES AT

PawsForTheGoodStuff.com/GetCurious

Watch my exclusive short video and discover how you
can take your journaling experience to the next level.

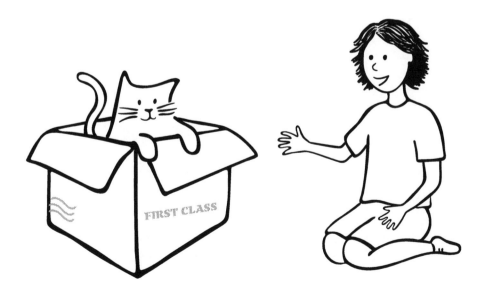

I believe cats to be spirits come to earth.
A cat, I am sure, could walk on a cloud without coming through.

JULES VERNE

Date _____

My *Pawsitive* Power Word of the Day _____

am

This morning I woke up feeling _____

As I go through my day I wish to feel _____

I am grateful to my cat, _____ because _____

How can my kitty BFF inspire me to have a more *pawsitive* day? (If you get stuck, use your power word.)

_____

pm

3 *pawsitive* things that happened to me today were...

🐾 _____

🐾 _____

🐾 _____

Tonight as I drift off to sleep I will send happiness & *pawsitive* thoughts to...

_____

It's the moments that I stopped just to be, rather than do,
that have given me true happiness.

RICHARD BRANSON

Date _____

My *Pawsitive* Power Word of the Day _____

am

This morning I woke up feeling _____

As I go through my day I wish to feel_____

I am grateful to my cat, _____ because _____

How can my kitty BFF inspire me to have a more *pawsitive* day? (If you get stuck, use your power word.)

_____

pm

3 *pawsitive* things that happened to me today were...

🐾 _____

🐾 _____

🐾 _____

Tonight as I drift off to sleep I will send happiness & *pawsitive* thoughts to...

_____

I had been told that the training procedure with cats was difficult.
It's not.Mine had me trained in two days.

BILL DANA

Date _____

My *Pawsitive* Power Word of the Day _____

am

This morning I woke up feeling _____

As I go through my day I wish to feel _____

I am grateful to my cat, _____ because _____

How can my kitty BFF inspire me to have a more *pawsitive* day? (If you get stuck, use your power word.)

pm

3 *pawsitive* things that happened to me today were...

🐾 _____

🐾 _____

🐾 _____

Tonight as I drift off to sleep I will send happiness & *pawsitive* thoughts to...

There is only one happiness in this life, to love and be loved.

GEORGE SAND

Date _____

My *Pawsitive* Power Word of the Day _____

am

This morning I woke up feeling _____

As I go through my day I wish to feel _____

I am grateful to my cat, _____ because _____

How can my kitty BFF inspire me to have a more *pawsitive* day? (If you get stuck, use your power word.)

_____

pm

3 *pawsitive* things that happened to me today were...

🐾 _____

🐾 _____

🐾 _____

Tonight as I drift off to sleep I will send happiness & *pawsitive* thoughts to...

_____

A true cat lover cradles a cat and knows that nine lives will never be nearly enough.

AUTHOR UNKNOWN

Date _____

My *Pawsitive* Power Word of the Day _____

am

This morning I woke up feeling _____

As I go through my day I wish to feel _____

I am grateful to my cat, _____ because _____

How can my kitty BFF inspire me to have a more *pawsitive* day? (If you get stuck, use your power word.)

_____

pm

3 *pawsitive* things that happened to me today were...

🐾 _____

🐾 _____

🐾 _____

Tonight as I drift off to sleep I will send happiness & *pawsitive* thoughts to...

_____

In a gentle way, you can shake the world.

MAHATMA GANDHI

Date _____

My *Pawsitive* Power Word of the Day _____

am

This morning I woke up feeling _____

As I go through my day I wish to feel _____

I am grateful to my cat, _____ because _____

How can my kitty BFF inspire me to have a more *pawsitive* day? (If you get stuck, use your power word.)

pm

3 *pawsitive* things that happened to me today were...

🐾 _____

🐾 _____

🐾 _____

Tonight as I drift off to sleep I will send happiness & *pawsitive* thoughts to...

I have lived with several Zen masters — all of them cats.

ECKHART TOLLE

The Seventh Day Challenge

What *Pawsitive Power word* resonates strongly with you?
Use it to create a personal affirmation. An affirmation is a powerful and positive
statement that you repeat such as, "I am healthy, I am happy, I am extraordinary!"
Use your affirmation regularly and whole-heartedly, and get ready to feel
even more *pawsitivity*!

Pawsitive Power Word

Affirmation

I believe that if one always looked at the skies, one would end up with wings.

GUSTAVE FLAUBERT

Date _____

My *Pawsitive* Power Word of the Day _____

am

This morning I woke up feeling _____

As I go through my day I wish to feel_____

I am grateful to my cat, _____ because _____

How can my kitty BFF inspire me to have a more *pawsitive* day? (If you get stuck, use your power word.)

pm

3 *pawsitive* things that happened to me today were...

🐾 _____

🐾 _____

🐾 _____

Tonight as I drift off to sleep I will send happiness & *pawsitive* thoughts to...

When I am feeling low all I have to do is watch my cats and my courage returns.

CHARLES BUKOWSKI

Date _____

My *Pawsitive* Power Word of the Day _____

am

This morning I woke up feeling _____

As I go through my day I wish to feel _____

I am grateful to my cat, _____ because _____

How can my kitty BFF inspire me to have a more *pawsitive* day? (If you get stuck, use your power word.)

_____

pm

3 *pawsitive* things that happened to me today were...

🐾 _____

🐾 _____

🐾 _____

Tonight as I drift off to sleep I will send happiness & *pawsitive* thoughts to...

_____

Optimism is the one quality more associated with success and happiness than any other.

BRIAN TRACY

Date _____

My *Pawsitive* Power Word of the Day _____

am

This morning I woke up feeling _____

As I go through my day I wish to feel _____

I am grateful to my cat, _____ because _____

How can my kitty BFF inspire me to have a more *pawsitive* day? (If you get stuck, use your power word.)

_____

pm

3 *pawsitive* things that happened to me today were...

🐾 _____

🐾 _____

🐾 _____

Tonight as I drift off to sleep I will send happiness & *pawsitive* thoughts to...

_____

Kittens are angels with whiskers.

ALEXIS FLORA HOPE

Date _____

My *Pawsitive* Power Word of the Day _____

am

This morning I woke up feeling _____

As I go through my day I wish to feel _____

I am grateful to my cat, _____ because _____

How can my kitty BFF inspire me to have a more *pawsitive* day? (If you get stuck, use your power word.)

pm

3 *pawsitive* things that happened to me today were...

🐾 _____

🐾 _____

🐾 _____

Tonight as I drift off to sleep I will send happiness & *pawsitive* thoughts to...

Do it with passion, or not at all.

ROSA NOUCHETTE CAREY

Date _____

My *Pawsitive* Power Word of the Day _____

am

This morning I woke up feeling _____

As I go through my day I wish to feel _____

I am grateful to my cat, _____ because _____

How can my kitty BFF inspire me to have a more *pawsitive* day? (If you get stuck, use your power word.)

_____

pm

3 *pawsitive* things that happened to me today were...

🐾 _____

🐾 _____

🐾 _____

Tonight as I drift off to sleep I will send happiness & *pawsitive* thoughts to...

_____

*Are we really sure the purring is coming from the kitty
and not from our very own hearts?*

TERRI GUILLEMETS

Date _____

My *Pawsitive* Power Word of the Day _____

am

This morning I woke up feeling _____

As I go through my day I wish to feel _____

I am grateful to my cat, _____ because _____

How can my kitty BFF inspire me to have a more *pawsitive* day? (If you get stuck, use your power word.)

pm

3 *pawsitive* things that happened to me today were...

🐾 _____

🐾 _____

🐾 _____

Tonight as I drift off to sleep I will send happiness & *pawsitive* thoughts to...

A No. 2 pencil and a dream can take you anywhere.

JOYCE MEYER

The Seventh Day Challenge

How does your cat inspire you to live your best life?

To err is human, to purr is feline.
ROBERT BYRNE

Did you know?

We cats are good for your health.

Research shows living with a cat can reduce your risk of stroke and heart attack by one third. We also excel at helping you let go of stress, anxiety, loneliness, and depression.

Love can heal any heart — and we have plenty of that to give you.

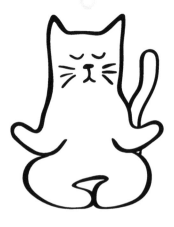

Life is not always a matter of holding good cards,
but sometimes, playing a poor hand well.

JACK LONDON

Date _____

My *Pawsitive* Power Word of the Day _____

am

This morning I woke up feeling _____

As I go through my day I wish to feel_____

I am grateful to my cat, _____ because _____

How can my kitty BFF inspire me to have a more *pawsitive* day? (If you get stuck, use your power word.)

_____

pm

3 *pawsitive* things that happened to me today were...

🐾 _____

🐾 _____

🐾 _____

Tonight as I drift off to sleep I will send happiness & *pawsitive* thoughts to...

_____

If a cat spoke, it would say things like 'Hey, I don't see the problem here'.
ROY BLOUNT JR.

Date _____

My *Pawsitive* Power Word of the Day _____

am

This morning I woke up feeling _____

As I go through my day I wish to feel _____

I am grateful to my cat, _____ because _____

How can my kitty BFF inspire me to have a more *pawsitive* day? (If you get stuck, use your power word.)

_____

pm

3 *pawsitive* things that happened to me today were...

🐾 _____

🐾 _____

🐾 _____

Tonight as I drift off to sleep I will send happiness & *pawsitive* thoughts to...

_____

Doing what you like is freedom. Liking what you do is happiness.

FRANK TYGER

Date _____

My *Pawsitive* Power Word of the Day _____

am

This morning I woke up feeling _____

As I go through my day I wish to feel _____

I am grateful to my cat, _____ because _____

How can my kitty BFF inspire me to have a more *pawsitive* day? (If you get stuck, use your power word.)

_____

pm

3 *pawsitive* things that happened to me today were...

🐾 _____

🐾 _____

🐾 _____

Tonight as I drift off to sleep I will send happiness & *pawsitive* thoughts to...

_____

The dog may be wonderful prose, but only the cat is poetry.

FRENCH PROVERB

Date _____

My *Pawsitive* Power Word of the Day _____

am

This morning I woke up feeling _____

As I go through my day I wish to feel _____

I am grateful to my cat, _____ because _____

How can my kitty BFF inspire me to have a more *pawsitive* day? (If you get stuck, use your power word.)

_____

pm

3 *pawsitive* things that happened to me today were...

🐾 _____

🐾 _____

🐾 _____

Tonight as I drift off to sleep I will send happiness & *pawsitive* thoughts to...

_____

The grass is greener where you water it.

NEIL BARRINGHAM

Date _____

My *Pawsitive* Power Word of the Day _____

am

This morning I woke up feeling _____

As I go through my day I wish to feel _____

I am grateful to my cat, _____ because _____

How can my kitty BFF inspire me to have a more *pawsitive* day? (If you get stuck, use your power word.)

pm

3 *pawsitive* things that happened to me today were...

🐾 _____

🐾 _____

🐾 _____

Tonight as I drift off to sleep I will send happiness & *pawsitive* thoughts to...

Dogs own space and cats own time.

NICOLA GRIFFITH, HILD

Date _____

My *Pawsitive* Power Word of the Day _____

am

This morning I woke up feeling _____

As I go through my day I wish to feel _____

I am grateful to my cat, _____ because _____

How can my kitty BFF inspire me to have a more *pawsitive* day? (If you get stuck, use your power word.)

_____

pm

3 *pawsitive* things that happened to me today were...

🐾 _____

🐾 _____

🐾 _____

Tonight as I drift off to sleep I will send happiness & *pawsitive* thoughts to...

_____

Life is 10% what happens to me and 90% of how I react to it.

CHARLES SWINDOLL

The Seventh Day Challenge

What do you think your cat is feeling right now?
What are you feeling in this moment?

*There is truly not a single quality of the cat
that man should not seek to emulate to improve.*

CARL VAN VECHTEN

Date _____

My *Pawsitive* Power Word of the Day _____

am

This morning I woke up feeling _____

As I go through my day I wish to feel _____

I am grateful to my cat, _____ because _____

How can my kitty BFF inspire me to have a more *pawsitive* day? (If you get stuck, use your power word.)

_____

pm

3 *pawsitive* things that happened to me today were...

🐾 _____

🐾 _____

🐾 _____

Tonight as I drift off to sleep I will send happiness & *pawsitive* thoughts to...

_____

If you look at what you have in life, you'll always have more.
If you look at what you don't have in life, you'll never have enough.

OPRAH WINFREY

Date _____

My *Pawsitive* Power Word of the Day _____

am

This morning I woke up feeling _____

As I go through my day I wish to feel _____

I am grateful to my cat, _____ because _____

How can my kitty BFF inspire me to have a more *pawsitive* day? (If you get stuck, use your power word.)

_____

pm

3 *pawsitive* things that happened to me today were...

🐾 _____

🐾 _____

🐾 _____

Tonight as I drift off to sleep I will send happiness & *pawsitive* thoughts to...

_____

Human beings are drawn to cats because they are all we are not — self-contained, elegant in everything they do, relaxed, assured, glad of company, yet still possessing secret lives.

PAM BROWN

Date _____

My *Pawsitive* Power Word of the Day _____

am

This morning I woke up feeling _____

As I go through my day I wish to feel _____

I am grateful to my cat, _____ because _____

How can my kitty BFF inspire me to have a more *pawsitive* day? (If you get stuck, use your power word.)

pm

3 *pawsitive* things that happened to me today were...

🐾 _____

🐾 _____

🐾 _____

Tonight as I drift off to sleep I will send happiness & *pawsitive* thoughts to...

Too many of us are not living our dreams because we are living our fears.

LES BROWN

Date _____

My *Pawsitive* Power Word of the Day _____

am

This morning I woke up feeling _____

As I go through my day I wish to feel _____

I am grateful to my cat, _____ because _____

How can my kitty BFF inspire me to have a more *pawsitive* day? (If you get stuck, use your power word.)

_____

pm

3 *pawsitive* things that happened to me today were...

🐾 _____

🐾 _____

🐾 _____

Tonight as I drift off to sleep I will send happiness & *pawsitive* thoughts to...

_____

You cannot ask for more if you are having a cat to love you unconditionally.

CHARLES DICKENS

Date _____

My *Pawsitive* Power Word of the Day _____

am

This morning I woke up feeling _____

As I go through my day I wish to feel _____

I am grateful to my cat, _____ because _____

How can my kitty BFF inspire me to have a more *pawsitive* day? (If you get stuck, use your power word.)

_____

pm

3 *pawsitive* things that happened to me today were...

🐾 _____

🐾 _____

🐾 _____

Tonight as I drift off to sleep I will send happiness & *pawsitive* thoughts to...

_____

Today is life — the only life you are sure of. Make the most of today.
Get interested in something. Shake yourself awake. Develop a hobby.
Let the winds of enthusiasm sweep through you. Live today with gusto.

DALE CARNEGIE

Date _____

My *Pawsitive* Power Word of the Day _____

am

This morning I woke up feeling _____

As I go through my day I wish to feel _____

I am grateful to my cat, _____ because _____

How can my kitty BFF inspire me to have a more *pawsitive* day? (If you get stuck, use your power word.)

_____

pm

3 *pawsitive* things that happened to me today were...

🐾 _____

🐾 _____

🐾 _____

Tonight as I drift off to sleep I will send happiness & *pawsitive* thoughts to...

_____

The Pawsitive Monthly Milestone

Give Your BFF a Gift!

Visit a pet store and pick up a little something for your furry friend.
On a budget? Not problem. Get creative and make something instead. Look online for
ideas —you won't believe what you can make from an empty toilet paper roll.
Take a picture of your BFF's reaction.

Place your picture below

#PawsForTheGoodStuff 🐾 Spread the *Pawsitivity*!

Share your picture with your online community and use #PawsForTheGoodStuff.
Together we can change the world, one *pawsitive* moment at a time.

Get Curious!

How Does it Feel?

Last month you added the elements of sight, sound, smell, touch, and taste to create a richer journaling experience. Shall we take it up another notch? You can do that by getting out of your head and into your heart.

LEARN MORE ON HOW IT FEELS AT

PawsForTheGoodStuff.com/GetCurious

Watch my exclusive short video and discover how you can take your journaling experience to the next level.

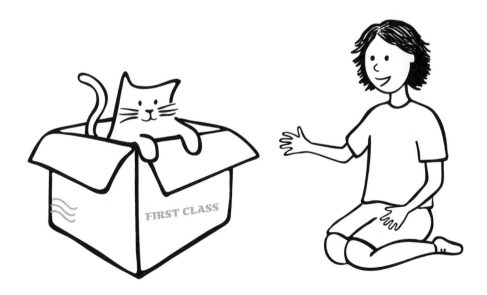

A kitten is, in the animal world, what a rosebud is in the garden.

ROBERT SOWTHEY

Date _____

My *Pawsitive* Power Word of the Day _____

am

This morning I woke up feeling _____

As I go through my day I wish to feel _____

I am grateful to my cat, _____ because _____

How can my kitty BFF inspire me to have a more *pawsitive* day? (If you get stuck, use your power word.)

_____

pm

3 *pawsitive* things that happened to me today were...

🐾 _____

🐾 _____

🐾 _____

Tonight as I drift off to sleep I will send happiness & *pawsitive* thoughts to...

_____

Change your thoughts and you change your world.

NORMAN VINCENT PEALE

Date _____

My *Pawsitive* Power Word of the Day _____

am

This morning I woke up feeling _____

As I go through my day I wish to feel_____

I am grateful to my cat, _____because _____

How can my kitty BFF inspire me to have a more *pawsitive* day? (If you get stuck, use your power word.)

_____

pm

3 *pawsitive* things that happened to me today were...

🐾 _____

🐾 _____

🐾 _____

Tonight as I drift off to sleep I will send happiness & *pawsitive* thoughts to...

_____

I realized that cats make a perfect audience, they don't laugh at you,
they never contradict you, there's no need to impress them,
and they won't divulge your secrets.

ELLE NEWMARK

Date _____

My *Pawsitive* Power Word of the Day _____

am

This morning I woke up feeling _____

As I go through my day I wish to feel _____

I am grateful to my cat, _____ because _____

How can my kitty BFF inspire me to have a more *pawsitive* day? (If you get stuck, use your power word.)

pm

3 *pawsitive* things that happened to me today were...

🐾 _____

🐾 _____

🐾 _____

Tonight as I drift off to sleep I will send happiness & *pawsitive* thoughts to...

Coming home to a wagging tail is the best part of the day.

P.C.CAST

Date _____

My *Pawsitive* Power Word of the Day _____

am

This morning I woke up feeling _____

As I go through my day I wish to feel_____

I am grateful to my cat, _____ because _____

How can my kitty BFF inspire me to have a more *pawsitive* day? (If you get stuck, use your power word.)

_____

pm

3 *pawsitive* things that happened to me today were...

🐾 _____

🐾 _____

🐾 _____

Tonight as I drift off to sleep I will send happiness & *pawsitive* thoughts to...

_____

The cat does not offer services. The cat offers itself.

WILLIAM S. BURROUGHS

Date _____

My *Pawsitive* Power Word of the Day _____

am

This morning I woke up feeling _____

As I go through my day I wish to feel _____

I am grateful to my cat, _____ because _____

How can my kitty BFF inspire me to have a more *pawsitive* day? (If you get stuck, use your power word.)

pm

3 *pawsitive* things that happened to me today were...

🐾 _____

🐾 _____

🐾 _____

Tonight as I drift off to sleep I will send happiness & *pawsitive* thoughts to...

Out of difficulties grow miracles.

JEAN DE LA BRUYERE

Date _____

My *Pawsitive* Power Word of the Day _____

am

This morning I woke up feeling _____

As I go through my day I wish to feel _____

I am grateful to my cat, _____ because _____

How can my kitty BFF inspire me to have a more *pawsitive* day? (If you get stuck, use your power word.)

_____

pm

3 *pawsitive* things that happened to me today were...

🐾 _____

🐾 _____

🐾 _____

Tonight as I drift off to sleep I will send happiness & *pawsitive* thoughts to...

_____

Way down deep, we're all motivated by the same urges.
Cats have the courage to live by them.

JIM DAVIS

The Seventh Day Challenge

Describe your favorite memory with your BFF.

Everything has beauty, but not everyone can see.

CONFUCIUS

Date _____

My *Pawsitive* Power Word of the Day _____

am

This morning I woke up feeling _____

As I go through my day I wish to feel _____

I am grateful to my cat, _____ because _____

How can my kitty BFF inspire me to have a more *pawsitive* day? (If you get stuck, use your power word.)

_____

pm

3 *pawsitive* things that happened to me today were...

🐾 _____

🐾 _____

🐾 _____

Tonight as I drift off to sleep I will send happiness & *pawsitive* thoughts to...

_____

I have felt cats rubbing their faces against mine and touching my cheek
with claws carefully sheathed. These things, to me, are expressions of love.

JAMES HERRIOT

Date _____

My *Pawsitive* Power Word of the Day _____

am

This morning I woke up feeling _____

As I go through my day I wish to feel _____

I am grateful to my cat, _____ because _____

How can my kitty BFF inspire me to have a more *pawsitive* day? (If you get stuck, use your power word.)

pm

3 *pawsitive* things that happened to me today were...

🐾 _____

🐾 _____

🐾 _____

Tonight as I drift off to sleep I will send happiness & *pawsitive* thoughts to...

When I was 5 years old, my mother always told me that happiness was the key to life.
When I went to school, they asked me what I wanted to be when I grew up. I wrote down 'happy.'
They told me I didn't understand the assignment, and I told them they didn't understand life.

JOHN LENNON

Date _____

My *Pawsitive* Power Word of the Day _____

am

This morning I woke up feeling _____

As I go through my day I wish to feel _____

I am grateful to my cat, _____ because _____

How can my kitty BFF inspire me to have a more *pawsitive* day? (If you get stuck, use your power word.)

_____

pm

3 *pawsitive* things that happened to me today were...

🐾 _____

🐾 _____

🐾 _____

Tonight as I drift off to sleep I will send happiness & *pawsitive* thoughts to...

_____

How we behave toward cats here below determines our status in heaven.

ROBERT A. HEINLEIN

Date _____

My *Pawsitive* Power Word of the Day _____

am

This morning I woke up feeling _____

As I go through my day I wish to feel _____

I am grateful to my cat, _____ because _____

How can my kitty BFF inspire me to have a more *pawsitive* day? (If you get stuck, use your power word.)

pm

3 *pawsitive* things that happened to me today were...

🐾 _____

🐾 _____

🐾 _____

Tonight as I drift off to sleep I will send happiness & *pawsitive* thoughts to...

The only person you are destined to become is the person you decide to be.

RALPH WALDO EMERSON

Date _____

My *Pawsitive* Power Word of the Day _____

am

This morning I woke up feeling _____

As I go through my day I wish to feel _____

I am grateful to my cat, _____ because _____

How can my kitty BFF inspire me to have a more *pawsitive* day? (If you get stuck, use your power word.)

pm

3 *pawsitive* things that happened to me today were...

🐾 _____

🐾 _____

🐾 _____

Tonight as I drift off to sleep I will send happiness & *pawsitive* thoughts to...

I regard cats as one of the great joys in the world. I see them as a gift of highest orders.

TRISHA MCCAGH

Date _____

My *Pawsitive* Power Word of the Day _____

am

This morning I woke up feeling _____

As I go through my day I wish to feel _____

I am grateful to my cat, _____ because _____

How can my kitty BFF inspire me to have a more *pawsitive* day? (If you get stuck, use your power word.)

pm

3 *pawsitive* things that happened to me today were...

🐾 _____

🐾 _____

🐾 _____

Tonight as I drift off to sleep I will send happiness & *pawsitive* thoughts to...

Who looks outside, dreams; who looks inside, awakes.

CARL JUNG

The Seventh Day Challenge

What stands between you and your joy?
How can your special connection to your kitty inspire you
to live a more *pawsitive* life?

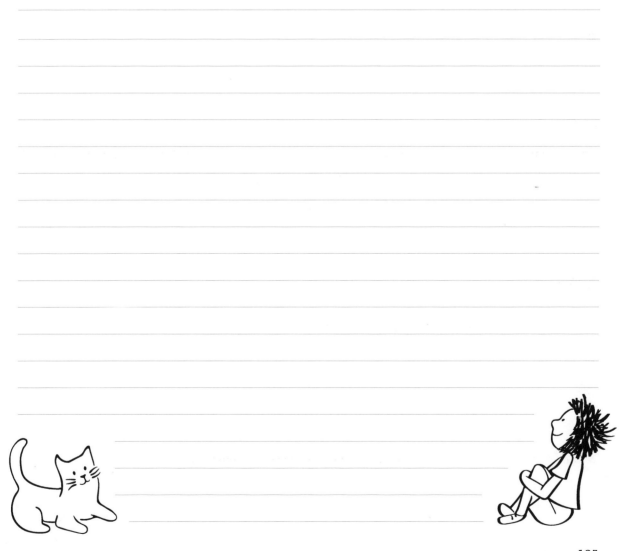

Did you know?

Our purrrrrrr is the cat's pajamas.

A purr does not just mean we are happy. Purring can also mean we are hungry or even in pain. We also purr to help ourselves heal. A cat purrs at a frequency of 25 to 150 Hertz. the frequency at which muscles and bones repair themselves.

And that ain't no hairball!

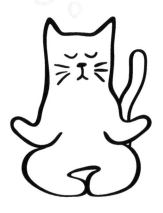

Difficult roads often lead to beautiful destinations.

WILLIAM ARTHUR WARD

Date _____

My *Pawsitive* Power Word of the Day _____

am

This morning I woke up feeling _____

As I go through my day I wish to feel _____

I am grateful to my cat, _____ because _____

How can my kitty BFF inspire me to have a more *pawsitive* day? (If you get stuck, use your power word.)

_____

pm

3 *pawsitive* things that happened to me today were...

🐾 _____

🐾 _____

🐾 _____

Tonight as I drift off to sleep I will send happiness & *pawsitive* thoughts to...

_____

My sunshine comes from the love in my cat's eyes.

CHRISTOPHER HITCHENS

Date _____

My *Pawsitive* Power Word of the Day _____

am

This morning I woke up feeling _____

As I go through my day I wish to feel _____

I am grateful to my cat, _____ because _____

How can my kitty BFF inspire me to have a more *pawsitive* day? (If you get stuck, use your power word.)

pm

3 *pawsitive* things that happened to me today were...

🐾 _____

🐾 _____

🐾 _____

Tonight as I drift off to sleep I will send happiness & *pawsitive* thoughts to...

A loving heart is the truest wisdom.

CHARLES DICKENS

Date _____

My *Pawsitive* Power Word of the Day _____

am

This morning I woke up feeling _____

As I go through my day I wish to feel _____

I am grateful to my cat, _____ because _____

How can my kitty BFF inspire me to have a more *pawsitive* day? (If you get stuck, use your power word.)

pm

3 *pawsitive* things that happened to me today were...

🐾 _____

🐾 _____

🐾 _____

Tonight as I drift off to sleep I will send happiness & *pawsitive* thoughts to...

The vibrations you receive when the cat purrs on your lap
are of contentment and pure love.

ST. FRANCIS OF ASSISI

Date _____

My *Pawsitive* Power Word of the Day _____

am

This morning I woke up feeling _____

As I go through my day I wish to feel _____

I am grateful to my cat, _____ because _____

How can my kitty BFF inspire me to have a more *pawsitive* day? (If you get stuck, use your power word.)

pm

3 *pawsitive* things that happened to me today were...

🐾 _____

🐾 _____

🐾 _____

Tonight as I drift off to sleep I will send happiness & *pawsitive* thoughts to...

130

Be happy. It really annoys negative people.

RICKY GERVAIS

Date _____

My *Pawsitive* Power Word of the Day _____

am

This morning I woke up feeling _____

As I go through my day I wish to feel _____

I am grateful to my cat, _____ because _____

How can my kitty BFF inspire me to have a more *pawsitive* day? (If you get stuck, use your power word.)

_____

pm

3 *pawsitive* things that happened to me today were...

🐾 _____

🐾 _____

🐾 _____

Tonight as I drift off to sleep I will send happiness & *pawsitive* thoughts to...

_____

Cats are a mysterious kind of folk.
There is more passing in their minds than we are aware of.

SIR WALTER SCOTT

Date _____

My *Pawsitive* Power Word of the Day _____

am

This morning I woke up feeling _____

As I go through my day I wish to feel _____

I am grateful to my cat, _____ because _____

How can my kitty BFF inspire me to have a more *pawsitive* day? (If you get stuck, use your power word.)

pm

3 *pawsitive* things that happened to me today were...

🐾 _____

🐾 _____

🐾 _____

Tonight as I drift off to sleep I will send happiness & *pawsitive* thoughts to...

Although the world is full of suffering, it is also full of the overcoming of it.

HELEN KELLER

The Seventh Day Challenge

List 10 things (besides your cat) that make you smile.
Remember to look at this "Happy List" anytime you are feeling blue.

1

2

3

4

5

6

7

8

9

10

God made the cat to give man the pleasure of stroking a tiger.

FRANCOIS JOSEPH MERY

Date _____

My *Pawsitive* Power Word of the Day _____

am

This morning I woke up feeling _____

As I go through my day I wish to feel _____

I am grateful to my cat, _____ because _____

How can my kitty BFF inspire me to have a more *pawsitive* day? (If you get stuck, use your power word.)

_____

pm

3 *pawsitive* things that happened to me today were...

🐾 _____

🐾 _____

🐾 _____

Tonight as I drift off to sleep I will send happiness & *pawsitive* thoughts to...

_____

Be yourself; everyone else is already taken.

OSCAR WILDE

Date _____

My *Pawsitive* Power Word of the Day _____

am

This morning I woke up feeling _____

As I go through my day I wish to feel _____

I am grateful to my cat, _____ because _____

How can my kitty BFF inspire me to have a more *pawsitive* day? (If you get stuck, use your power word.)

pm

3 *pawsitive* things that happened to me today were...

🐾 _____

🐾 _____

🐾 _____

Tonight as I drift off to sleep I will send happiness & *pawsitive* thoughts to...

Dogs come when they're called; cats take a message and get back to you later.

MARY BLY

Date _____

My *Pawsitive* Power Word of the Day _____

am

This morning I woke up feeling _____

As I go through my day I wish to feel _____

I am grateful to my cat, _____ because _____

How can my kitty BFF inspire me to have a more *pawsitive* day? (If you get stuck, use your power word.)

pm

3 *pawsitive* things that happened to me today were...

🐾 _____

🐾 _____

🐾 _____

Tonight as I drift off to sleep I will send happiness & *pawsitive* thoughts to...

Magic is believing in yourself, if you can do that, you can make anything happen.

JOHANN WOLFGANG VON GOETHE

Date _____

My *Pawsitive* Power Word of the Day _____

am

This morning I woke up feeling _____

As I go through my day I wish to feel _____

I am grateful to my cat, _____ because _____

How can my kitty BFF inspire me to have a more *pawsitive* day? (If you get stuck, use your power word.)

_____

pm

3 *pawsitive* things that happened to me today were...

🐾 _____

🐾 _____

🐾 _____

Tonight as I drift off to sleep I will send happiness & *pawsitive* thoughts to...

_____

In the middle of a world that had always been a bit mad, the cat walks with confidence.

ROSANNE AMBERSON

Date _____

My *Pawsitive* Power Word of the Day _____

am

This morning I woke up feeling _____

As I go through my day I wish to feel _____

I am grateful to my cat, _____ because _____

How can my kitty BFF inspire me to have a more *pawsitive* day? (If you get stuck, use your power word.)

pm

3 *pawsitive* things that happened to me today were...

🐾 _____

🐾 _____

🐾 _____

Tonight as I drift off to sleep I will send happiness & *pawsitive* thoughts to...

*Three grand essentials to happiness in this life are something to do,
something to love, and something to hope for.*

JOSEPH ADDISON

Date _____

My *Pawsitive* Power Word of the Day _____

am

This morning I woke up feeling _____

As I go through my day I wish to feel _____

I am grateful to my cat, _____ because _____

How can my kitty BFF inspire me to have a more *pawsitive* day? (If you get stuck, use your power word.)

_____

pm

3 *pawsitive* things that happened to me today were...

🐾 _____

🐾 _____

🐾 _____

Tonight as I drift off to sleep I will send happiness & *pawsitive* thoughts to...

_____

The Pawsitive Monthly Milestone

Expand Your Imagination!

Curl up in bed and read your favorite book — to your cat.
Cats feel comforted when their guardian reads aloud to them - or at least that's what
people who have read *Dog as My Doctor, Cat as My Nurse* have told me. Not much of
a reader? Try watching cat videos on YouTube, or singing to your cat. The point is to
enjoy some quality time together. Take a selfie to remember the moment.

Place your selfie below

#PawsForTheGoodStuff 🐾 Spread the *Pawsitivity*!

Share your picture with your online community and use #PawsForTheGoodStuff.
Together we can change the world, one *pawsitive* moment at a time.

Get Curious!

Recognizing Resistance

Are you feeling happier, more cheerful, and generally more *pawsitive*? But are you also feeling lazy, bored, or struggling with your journal? If so, you may be experiencing *resistance*.

Resistance sneaks up in our relationships and careers, and side tracks us from our deepest desires. Learn to recognize and conquer your resistance.

LEARN MORE ON RECOGNIZING RESISTANCE AT

PawsForTheGoodStuff.com/GetCurious

Watch my exclusive short video and discover how you can take your journaling experience to the next level.

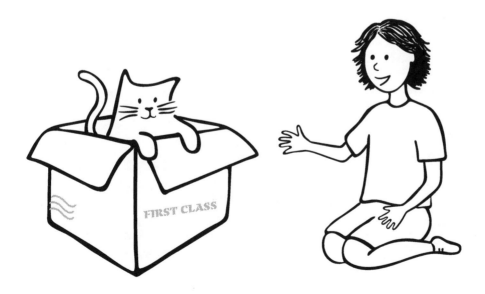

The cat was created when the lion sneezed.

ARABIAN PROVERB

Date _____

My *Pawsitive* Power Word of the Day _____

am

This morning I woke up feeling _____

As I go through my day I wish to feel _____

I am grateful to my cat, _____ because _____

How can my kitty BFF inspire me to have a more *pawsitive* day? (If you get stuck, use your power word.)

pm

3 *pawsitive* things that happened to me today were...

🐾 _____

🐾 _____

🐾 _____

Tonight as I drift off to sleep I will send happiness & *pawsitive* thoughts to...

Happiness is a butterfly, which when pursued, is always just beyond your grasp,
but which, if you will sit down quietly, may alight upon you.

NATHANIEL HAWTHORNE

Date _____

My *Pawsitive* Power Word of the Day _____

am

This morning I woke up feeling _____

As I go through my day I wish to feel _____

I am grateful to my cat, _____ because _____

How can my kitty BFF inspire me to have a more *pawsitive* day? (If you get stuck, use your power word.)

_____

pm

3 *pawsitive* things that happened to me today were...

🐾 _____

🐾 _____

🐾 _____

Tonight as I drift off to sleep I will send happiness & *pawsitive* thoughts to...

_____

*Cats are a tonic, they are a laugh, they are a cuddle, they are at least
pretty just about all of the time and beautiful some of the time.*

ROGER CARAS

Date _____

My *Pawsitive* Power Word of the Day _____

am

This morning I woke up feeling _____

As I go through my day I wish to feel _____

I am grateful to my cat, _____ because _____

How can my kitty BFF inspire me to have a more *pawsitive* day? (If you get stuck, use your power word.)

_____

pm

3 *pawsitive* things that happened to me today were...

🐾 _____

🐾 _____

🐾 _____

Tonight as I drift off to sleep I will send happiness & *pawsitive* thoughts to...

_____

The most common way people give up their power is by thinking they don't have any.

ALICE WALKER

Date _____

My *Pawsitive* Power Word of the Day _____

am

This morning I woke up feeling _____

As I go through my day I wish to feel_____

I am grateful to my cat, _____ because _____

How can my kitty BFF inspire me to have a more *pawsitive* day? (If you get stuck, use your power word.)

pm

3 *pawsitive* things that happened to me today were...

🐾 _____

🐾 _____

🐾 _____

Tonight as I drift off to sleep I will send happiness & *pawsitive* thoughts to...

Like a graceful vase, a cat, even when motionless, seems to flow.

GEORGE F. WILL

Date _____

My *Pawsitive* Power Word of the Day _____

am

This morning I woke up feeling _____

As I go through my day I wish to feel _____

I am grateful to my cat, _____ because _____

How can my kitty BFF inspire me to have a more *pawsitive* day? (If you get stuck, use your power word.)

pm

3 *pawsitive* things that happened to me today were...

🐾 _____

🐾 _____

🐾 _____

Tonight as I drift off to sleep I will send happiness & *pawsitive* thoughts to...

Happiness, not in another place but this place... not for another hour, but this hour.

WALT WHITMAN

Date _____

My *Pawsitive* Power Word of the Day _____

am

This morning I woke up feeling _____

As I go through my day I wish to feel _____

I am grateful to my cat, _____ because _____

How can my kitty BFF inspire me to have a more *pawsitive* day? (If you get stuck, use your power word.)

_____

pm

3 *pawsitive* things that happened to me today were...

🐾 _____

🐾 _____

🐾 _____

Tonight as I drift off to sleep I will send happiness & *pawsitive* thoughts to...

_____

Everything I know I learned from my cat: When you're hungry, eat.
When you're tired, nap in a sunbeam. When you go to the vet's, pee on your owner.

GARY SMITH

The Seventh Day Challenge

If your cat were your doctor, what advice would she/he give you?

People don't notice whether it's winter or summer when they're happy.

ANTON CHEKHOV

Date _____

My *Pawsitive* Power Word of the Day _____

am

This morning I woke up feeling _____

As I go through my day I wish to feel _____

I am grateful to my cat, _____ because _____

How can my kitty BFF inspire me to have a more *pawsitive* day? (If you get stuck, use your power word.)

_____

pm

3 *pawsitive* things that happened to me today were...

🐾 _____

🐾 _____

🐾 _____

Tonight as I drift off to sleep I will send happiness & *pawsitive* thoughts to...

_____

Cats choose us, we don't own them.

KRISTEN CAST

Date _____

My *Pawsitive* Power Word of the Day _____

am

This morning I woke up feeling _____

As I go through my day I wish to feel _____

I am grateful to my cat, _____ because _____

How can my kitty BFF inspire me to have a more *pawsitive* day? (If you get stuck, use your power word.)

pm

3 *pawsitive* things that happened to me today were...

🐾 _____

🐾 _____

🐾 _____

Tonight as I drift off to sleep I will send happiness & *pawsitive* thoughts to...

Of all the things you wear, your expression is the most important.

JANET LANE

Date _____

My *Pawsitive* Power Word of the Day _____

am

This morning I woke up feeling _____

As I go through my day I wish to feel _____

I am grateful to my cat, _____ because _____

How can my kitty BFF inspire me to have a more *pawsitive* day? (If you get stuck, use your power word.)

pm

3 *pawsitive* things that happened to me today were...

🐾 _____

🐾 _____

🐾 _____

Tonight as I drift off to sleep I will send happiness & *pawsitive* thoughts to...

To some blind souls all cats are much alike. To a cat lover every cat from the beginning of time has been utterly and amazingly unique.

JENNY DE VRIES

Date _____

My *Pawsitive* Power Word of the Day _____

am

This morning I woke up feeling _____

As I go through my day I wish to feel _____

I am grateful to my cat, _____ because _____

How can my kitty BFF inspire me to have a more *pawsitive* day? (If you get stuck, use your power word.)

_____

pm

3 *pawsitive* things that happened to me today were...

🐾 _____

🐾 _____

🐾 _____

Tonight as I drift off to sleep I will send happiness & *pawsitive* thoughts to...

_____

A truly happy person is one who can enjoy the scenery while on a detour.

GREGORY BENFORD

Date _____

My *Pawsitive* Power Word of the Day _____

am

This morning I woke up feeling _____

As I go through my day I wish to feel_____

I am grateful to my cat, _____ because _____

How can my kitty BFF inspire me to have a more *pawsitive* day? (If you get stuck, use your power word.)

pm

3 *pawsitive* things that happened to me today were...

🐾 _____

🐾 _____

🐾 _____

Tonight as I drift off to sleep I will send happiness & *pawsitive* thoughts to...

Cats own numerous charms which will make you forget all your worries.

SAKI

Date _____

My *Pawsitive* Power Word of the Day _____

am

This morning I woke up feeling _____

As I go through my day I wish to feel _____

I am grateful to my cat, _____ because _____

How can my kitty BFF inspire me to have a more *pawsitive* day? (If you get stuck, use your power word.)

_____

pm

3 *pawsitive* things that happened to me today were...

🐾 _____

🐾 _____

🐾 _____

Tonight as I drift off to sleep I will send happiness & *pawsitive* thoughts to...

_____

Now and then it's good to pause in our pursuit of happiness and just be happy.
GUILLAUME APOLLINAIRE

The Seventh Day Challenge

Draw anything you want on this page.
Use a pen, pencil, or try crayons — let your creativity soar!

No amount of time can erase the memory of a good cat, and no amount of masking tape can ever totally remove his fur from your couch.

LEO DWORKEN

Did you know?

You are never too old to play. Play fuels your imagination, stimulates your mind and makes you feel young. Just look at us! We love to chase a light, pounce at invisible monsters under the bedcovers, and pursue fluffy objects at the end of a string. Our advice? Play often, love lots, and purr with delight!

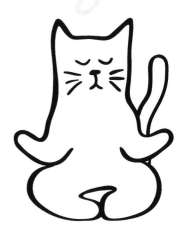

One happiness scatters a thousand sorrows.

CHINESE PROVERB

Date _____

My *Pawsitive* Power Word of the Day _____

am

This morning I woke up feeling _____

As I go through my day I wish to feel _____

I am grateful to my cat, _____ because _____

How can my kitty BFF inspire me to have a more *pawsitive* day? (If you get stuck, use your power word.)

_____

pm

3 *pawsitive* things that happened to me today were...

🐾 _____

🐾 _____

🐾 _____

Tonight as I drift off to sleep I will send happiness & *pawsitive* thoughts to...

_____

We need cats to need us. It unnerves us that they do not.
However, if they do not need us, they nonetheless seem to love us.

JEFFREY MOUSSAIEFF MASSON

Date _____

My *Pawsitive* Power Word of the Day _____

am

This morning I woke up feeling _____

As I go through my day I wish to feel _____

I am grateful to my cat, _____ because _____

How can my kitty BFF inspire me to have a more *pawsitive* day? (If you get stuck, use your power word.)

pm

3 *pawsitive* things that happened to me today were...

🐾 _____

🐾 _____

🐾 _____

Tonight as I drift off to sleep I will send happiness & *pawsitive* thoughts to...

When someone told me I lived in a fantasyland I nearly fell off my unicorn.
AUTHOR UNKNOWN

Date _____

My *Pawsitive* Power Word of the Day _____

am

This morning I woke up feeling _____

As I go through my day I wish to feel _____

I am grateful to my cat, _____ because _____

How can my kitty BFF inspire me to have a more *pawsitive* day? (If you get stuck, use your power word.)

_____

pm

3 *pawsitive* things that happened to me today were...

🐾 _____

🐾 _____

🐾 _____

Tonight as I drift off to sleep I will send happiness & *pawsitive* thoughts to...

_____

A best friend is like a four leaf clover, hard to find, lucky to have.

IRISH PROVERB

Date _____

My *Pawsitive* Power Word of the Day _____

am

This morning I woke up feeling _____

As I go through my day I wish to feel _____

I am grateful to my cat, _____ because _____

How can my kitty BFF inspire me to have a more *pawsitive* day? (If you get stuck, use your power word.)

_____

pm

3 *pawsitive* things that happened to me today were...

🐾 _____

🐾 _____

🐾 _____

Tonight as I drift off to sleep I will send happiness & *pawsitive* thoughts to...

_____

The best way to cheer yourself is to try to cheer someone else up.

MARK TWAIN

Date _____

My *Pawsitive* Power Word of the Day _____

am

This morning I woke up feeling _____

As I go through my day I wish to feel _____

I am grateful to my cat, _____ because _____

How can my kitty BFF inspire me to have a more *pawsitive* day? (If you get stuck, use your power word.)

_____

pm

3 *pawsitive* things that happened to me today were...

🐾 _____

🐾 _____

🐾 _____

Tonight as I drift off to sleep I will send happiness & *pawsitive* thoughts to...

_____

She clawed her way into my heart and wouldn't let go.

TERRI GUILLEMETS

Date _____

My *Pawsitive* Power Word of the Day _____

am

This morning I woke up feeling _____

As I go through my day I wish to feel _____

I am grateful to my cat, _____ because _____

How can my kitty BFF inspire me to have a more *pawsitive* day? (If you get stuck, use your power word.)

pm

3 *pawsitive* things that happened to me today were...

🐾 _____

🐾 _____

🐾 _____

Tonight as I drift off to sleep I will send happiness & *pawsitive* thoughts to...

Thousands of candles can be lit from a single candle, and the life of the candle
will not be shortened. Happiness never decreases by being shared.

GUATAMA BUDDHA

The Seventh Day Challenge

What is your cat's most unique quality?
What is your most unique quality?

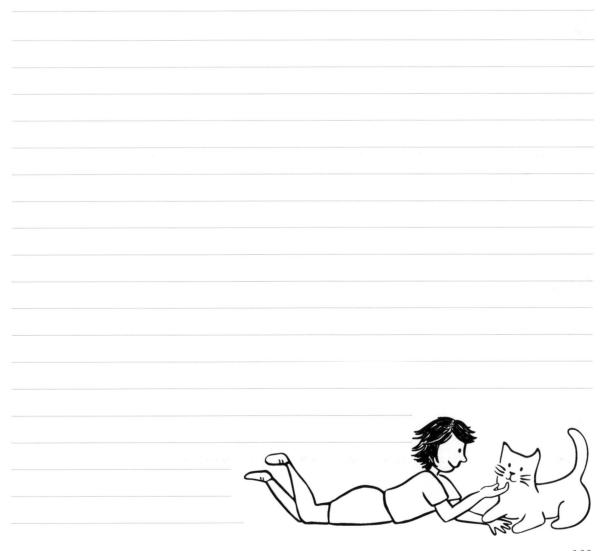

There are two means of refuge from the miseries of life: music and cats.

ALBERT SCHWEITZER

Date _____

My *Pawsitive* Power Word of the Day _____

am

This morning I woke up feeling _____

As I go through my day I wish to feel _____

I am grateful to my cat, _____ because _____

How can my kitty BFF inspire me to have a more *pawsitive* day? (If you get stuck, use your power word.)

pm

3 *pawsitive* things that happened to me today were...

🐾 _____

🐾 _____

🐾 _____

Tonight as I drift off to sleep I will send happiness & *pawsitive* thoughts to...

The biggest adventure you can take is to live the life of your dreams.

OPRAH WINFREY

Date _____

My *Pawsitive* Power Word of the Day _____

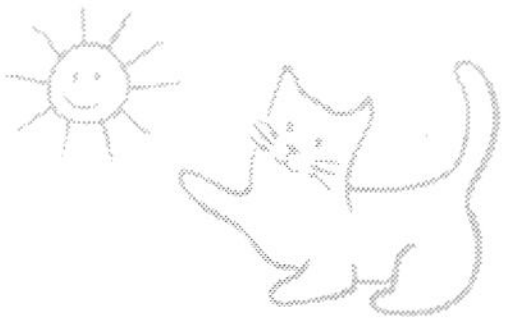

am

This morning I woke up feeling _____

As I go through my day I wish to feel _____

I am grateful to my cat, _____ because _____

How can my kitty BFF inspire me to have a more *pawsitive* day? (If you get stuck, use your power word.)

_____

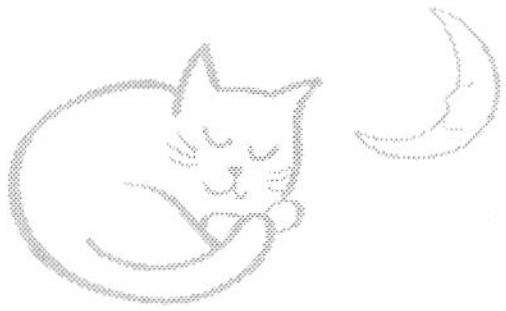

pm

3 *pawsitive* things that happened to me today were...

🐾 _____

🐾 _____

🐾 _____

Tonight as I drift off to sleep I will send happiness & *pawsitive* thoughts to...

_____

A cat improves the garden wall in sunshine, and the hearth in foul weather.

JUDITH MERKLE RILEY

Date _____

My *Pawsitive* Power Word of the Day _____

am

This morning I woke up feeling _____

As I go through my day I wish to feel _____

I am grateful to my cat, _____ because _____

How can my kitty BFF inspire me to have a more *pawsitive* day? (If you get stuck, use your power word.)

pm

3 *pawsitive* things that happened to me today were...

🐾 _____

🐾 _____

🐾 _____

Tonight as I drift off to sleep I will send happiness & *pawsitive* thoughts to...

Happiness does not lead to gratitude. Gratitude leads to happiness.
DAVID STEINDL-RAST

Date _____

My *Pawsitive* Power Word of the Day _____

am

This morning I woke up feeling _____

As I go through my day I wish to feel _____

I am grateful to my cat, _____ because _____

How can my kitty BFF inspire me to have a more *pawsitive* day? (If you get stuck, use your power word.)

pm

3 *pawsitive* things that happened to me today were...

🐾 _____

🐾 _____

🐾 _____

Tonight as I drift off to sleep I will send happiness & *pawsitive* thoughts to...

I put down my book, The Meaning of Zen, *and see the cat smiling into her fur*
as she delicately combs it with her rough pink tongue. 'Cat, I would lend you this book to study
but it appears you have already read it.' She looks up and gives me her full gaze.
'Don't be ridiculous,' she purrs, 'I wrote it.'

DILYS LAING

Date _____

My *Pawsitive* Power Word of the Day _____

am

This morning I woke up feeling _____

As I go through my day I wish to feel _____

I am grateful to my cat, _____ because _____

How can my kitty BFF inspire me to have a more *pawsitive* day? (If you get stuck, use your power word.)

_____

pm

3 *pawsitive* things that happened to me today were...

🐾 _____

🐾 _____

🐾 _____

Tonight as I drift off to sleep I will send happiness & *pawsitive* thoughts to...

_____

Life is short. Smile while you still have teeth.

MALLORY HOPKINS

Date _____

My *Pawsitive* Power Word of the Day _____

am

This morning I woke up feeling _____

As I go through my day I wish to feel _____

I am grateful to my cat, _____ because _____

How can my kitty BFF inspire me to have a more *pawsitive* day? (If you get stuck, use your power word.)

_____

pm

3 *pawsitive* things that happened to me today were...

🐾 _____

🐾 _____

🐾 _____

Tonight as I drift off to sleep I will send happiness & *pawsitive* thoughts to...

_____

The Pawsitive Monthly Milestone

Go Fetch!

Did you know cats enjoy a good game of fetch?
If you crumple a piece of paper and toss it across the room you will get a good chuckle watching your kitty make a mad dash to bring it back to you. It's great exercise for them and when they tire and you have to pick up the paper balls - it's a little exercise for you too! Don't forget to take pictures.

Place your favorite picture below

#PawsForTheGoodStuff 🐾 **Spread the *Pawsitivity*!**

Share your picture with your online community and use #PawsForTheGoodStuff.
Together we can change the world, one *pawsitive* moment at a time.

Get Curious!

Dig Deeper & Wider

Besides your cat, is there another animal that you feel grateful for?
A bird who sings at your window; an elephant whose strength you
admire; a cow whose gentle gaze has touched your heart? There are
many reasons to be grateful to all of the animals we share our amazing
world with. This month, focus on giving gratitude to other animals in
addition to your own.

LEARN MORE GO TO

PawsForTheGoodStuff.com/GetCurious

Watch my exclusive short video and discover how
to take your journaling experience to the next level.

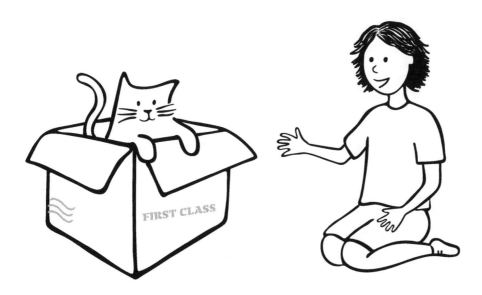

People who love cats have some of the biggest hearts around.
SUSAN EASTERLY

Date _____

My *Pawsitive* Power Word of the Day _____

am

This morning I woke up feeling _____

As I go through my day I wish to feel _____

I am grateful to my cat, _____ because _____

How can my kitty BFF inspire me to have a more *pawsitive* day? (If you get stuck, use your power word.)

pm

3 *pawsitive* things that happened to me today were...

🐾 _____

🐾 _____

🐾 _____

Tonight as I drift off to sleep I will send happiness & *pawsitive* thoughts to...

On the whole, the happiest people seem to be those
who have no particular cause for being happy except that they are so.

WILLIAM R. INGE

Date _____

My *Pawsitive* Power Word of the Day _____

am

This morning I woke up feeling _____

As I go through my day I wish to feel_____

I am grateful to my cat, _____ because _____

How can my kitty BFF inspire me to have a more *pawsitive* day? (If you get stuck, use your power word.)

_____

pm

3 *pawsitive* things that happened to me today were...

🐾 _____

🐾 _____

🐾 _____

Tonight as I drift off to sleep I will send happiness & *pawsitive* thoughts to...

_____

Who needs television when you have cats?

LORI SPIGELMYER

Date _____

My *Pawsitive* Power Word of the Day _____

am

This morning I woke up feeling _____

As I go through my day I wish to feel _____

I am grateful to my cat, _____ because _____

How can my kitty BFF inspire me to have a more *pawsitive* day? (If you get stuck, use your power word.)

pm

3 *pawsitive* things that happened to me today were...

- ❖ _____
- ❖ _____
- ❖ _____

Tonight as I drift off to sleep I will send happiness & *pawsitive* thoughts to...

Cry. Forgive. Learn. Move on. Let your tears water the seeds of your future happiness.

STEVE MARABOLI

Date _____

My *Pawsitive* Power Word of the Day _____

am

This morning I woke up feeling _____

As I go through my day I wish to feel _____

I am grateful to my cat, _____ because _____

How can my kitty BFF inspire me to have a more *pawsitive* day? (If you get stuck, use your power word.)

_____

pm

3 *pawsitive* things that happened to me today were...

🐾 _____

🐾 _____

🐾 _____

Tonight as I drift off to sleep I will send happiness & *pawsitive* thoughts to...

_____

Cats come and go without ever leaving.

MARTHA CURTIS

Date _____

My *Pawsitive* Power Word of the Day _____

am

This morning I woke up feeling _____

As I go through my day I wish to feel _____

I am grateful to my cat, _____ because _____

How can my kitty BFF inspire me to have a more *pawsitive* day? (If you get stuck, use your power word.)

pm

3 *pawsitive* things that happened to me today were...

🐾 _____

🐾 _____

🐾 _____

Tonight as I drift off to sleep I will send happiness & *pawsitive* thoughts to...

Happiness is the best makeup: a smile is better than any lipstick you'll put on.
DREW BARRYMORE

The Seventh Day Challenge

They say laughter is the best medicine.
What does your cat do to make you laugh?

Plenty of people miss their share of happiness, not because they never found it, but because they didn't stop to enjoy it.

WILLIAM FEATHER

Date _____

My *Pawsitive* Power Word of the Day _____

am

This morning I woke up feeling _____

As I go through my day I wish to feel _____

I am grateful to my cat, _____ because _____

How can my kitty BFF inspire me to have a more *pawsitive* day? (If you get stuck, use your power word.)

pm

3 *pawsitive* things that happened to me today were...

🐾 _____

🐾 _____

🐾 _____

Tonight as I drift off to sleep I will send happiness & *pawsitive* thoughts to...

Just because you are happy it does not mean that the day is perfect
but that you have looked beyond its imperfections.

BOB MARLEY

Date _____

My *Pawsitive* Power Word of the Day _____

am

This morning I woke up feeling _____

As I go through my day I wish to feel _____

I am grateful to my cat, _____ because _____

How can my kitty BFF inspire me to have a more *pawsitive* day? (If you get stuck, use your power word.)

pm

3 *pawsitive* things that happened to me today were...

🐾 _____

🐾 _____

🐾 _____

Tonight as I drift off to sleep I will send happiness & *pawsitive* thoughts to...

*It is impossible for a lover of cats to banish these alert, gentle, and discriminating friends,
who give us just enough of their regard and complaisance to make us hunger for more.*

AGNES REPPLIER

Did you know?

We may like the taste of milk but it doesn't like us back.

Like humans, cats aren't cows. So we often have trouble digesting lactose, a sugar present in milk. Drinking milk can lead to an upset tummy or worse. Try offering us some pumpkin puree instead. Our tummies like that.

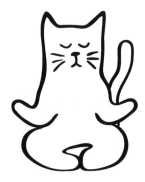

180

If we would just slow down, happiness would catch up to us.

RICHARD CARLS

Date _____

My *Pawsitive* Power Word of the Day _____

am

This morning I woke up feeling _____

As I go through my day I wish to feel _____

I am grateful to my cat, _____ because _____

How can my kitty BFF inspire me to have a more *pawsitive* day? (If you get stuck, use your power word.)

_____

pm

3 *pawsitive* things that happened to me today were...

🐾 _____

🐾 _____

🐾 _____

Tonight as I drift off to sleep I will send happiness & *pawsitive* thoughts to...

_____

You can not look at a sleeping cat and feel tense.

JANE PAULEY

Date _____

My *Pawsitive* Power Word of the Day _____

am

This morning I woke up feeling _____

As I go through my day I wish to feel _____

I am grateful to my cat, _____ because _____

How can my kitty BFF inspire me to have a more *pawsitive* day? (If you get stuck, use your power word.)

pm

3 *pawsitive* things that happened to me today were...

🐾 _____

🐾 _____

🐾 _____

Tonight as I drift off to sleep I will send happiness & *pawsitive* thoughts to...

Don't postpone joy until you have learned all of your lessons. Joy is your lesson.

ALAN COHEN

Date _____

My *Pawsitive* Power Word of the Day _____

am

This morning I woke up feeling _____

As I go through my day I wish to feel _____

I am grateful to my cat, _____ because _____

How can my kitty BFF inspire me to have a more *pawsitive* day? (If you get stuck, use your power word.)

_____

pm

3 *pawsitive* things that happened to me today were...

🐾 _____

🐾 _____

🐾 _____

Tonight as I drift off to sleep I will send happiness & *pawsitive* thoughts to...

_____

A cat has beauty without vanity, strength without insolence,
courage without ferocity, all the virtues of man without his vices.

LORD BYRON

Date _____

My *Pawsitive* Power Word of the Day _____

am

This morning I woke up feeling _____

As I go through my day I wish to feel _____

I am grateful to my cat, _____ because _____

How can my kitty BFF inspire me to have a more *pawsitive* day? (If you get stuck, use your power word.)

_____

pm

3 *pawsitive* things that happened to me today were...

🐾 _____

🐾 _____

🐾 _____

Tonight as I drift off to sleep I will send happiness & *pawsitive* thoughts to...

_____

The happiness of life is made up of the little charities of a kiss or smile,
a kind look, a heartfelt compliment.

SAMUEL TAYLOR COLERIDGE

The Seventh Day Challenge

Cats get excited over simple things — catnip, an empty box, a mysterious paper sack.
What gets you excited about life?

A kitten is the delight of a household.
All day long a comedy is played out by an incomparable actor.

CHAMPFLEURY

Date _____

My *Pawsitive* Power Word of the Day _____

am

This morning I woke up feeling _____

As I go through my day I wish to feel _____

I am grateful to my cat, _____ because _____

How can my kitty BFF inspire me to have a more *pawsitive* day? (If you get stuck, use your power word.)

_____

pm

3 *pawsitive* things that happened to me today were...

🐾 _____

🐾 _____

🐾 _____

Tonight as I drift off to sleep I will send happiness & *pawsitive* thoughts to...

_____

Happiness always looks small while you hold it in your hands,
but let it go, and you learn at once how big and precious it is.

MAXIM GORKY

Date _____

My *Pawsitive* Power Word of the Day _____

am

This morning I woke up feeling _____

As I go through my day I wish to feel_____

I am grateful to my cat, _____ because _____

How can my kitty BFF inspire me to have a more *pawsitive* day? (If you get stuck, use your power word.)

_____

pm

3 *pawsitive* things that happened to me today were...

🐾 _____

🐾 _____

🐾 _____

Tonight as I drift off to sleep I will send happiness & *pawsitive* thoughts to...

_____

Heaven will never be Paradise unless my cats are there waiting for me.

AUTHOR UNKNOWN

Date _____

My *Pawsitive* Power Word of the Day _____

am

This morning I woke up feeling _____

As I go through my day I wish to feel _____

I am grateful to my cat, _____ because _____

How can my kitty BFF inspire me to have a more *pawsitive* day? (If you get stuck, use your power word.)

_____

pm

3 *pawsitive* things that happened to me today were...

🐾 _____

🐾 _____

🐾 _____

Tonight as I drift off to sleep I will send happiness & *pawsitive* thoughts to...

_____

Light tomorrow with today.

ELIZABETH BARRETT BROWNING

Date _____

My *Pawsitive* Power Word of the Day _____

am

This morning I woke up feeling _____

As I go through my day I wish to feel _____

I am grateful to my cat, _____ because _____

How can my kitty BFF inspire me to have a more *pawsitive* day? (If you get stuck, use your power word.)

_____

pm

3 *pawsitive* things that happened to me today were...

🐾 _____

🐾 _____

🐾 _____

Tonight as I drift off to sleep I will send happiness & *pawsitive* thoughts to...

_____

I've found that the way a person feels about cats — and the way they feel about him or her in return — is usually an excellent gauge by which to measure a person's character.

P.C. CAST

Date _____

My *Pawsitive* Power Word of the Day _____

am

This morning I woke up feeling _____

As I go through my day I wish to feel _____

I am grateful to my cat, _____ because _____

How can my kitty BFF inspire me to have a more *pawsitive* day? (If you get stuck, use your power word.)

pm

3 *pawsitive* things that happened to me today were...

🐾 _____

🐾 _____

🐾 _____

Tonight as I drift off to sleep I will send happiness & *pawsitive* thoughts to...

To the mind that is still, the whole universe surrenders.

LAO TZU

Date _____

My *Pawsitive* Power Word of the Day _____

am

This morning I woke up feeling _____

As I go through my day I wish to feel _____

I am grateful to my cat, _____ because _____

How can my kitty BFF inspire me to have a more *pawsitive* day? (If you get stuck, use your power word.)

_____

pm

3 *pawsitive* things that happened to me today were...

🐾 _____

🐾 _____

🐾 _____

Tonight as I drift off to sleep I will send happiness & *pawsitive* thoughts to...

_____

In nine lifetimes, you'll never know as much about your cat
as your cat knows about you.

MICHEL DE MONTAIGNE

The Seventh Day Challenge

Become a cat.
Sit back and observe your kitty when they are in a state of simply *being*.
How does watching them be so peaceful and content feel to you?

Happiness is an inside job.

WILLIAM ARTHUR WARD

Date _____

My *Pawsitive* Power Word of the Day _____

am

This morning I woke up feeling _____

As I go through my day I wish to feel _____

I am grateful to my cat, _____ because _____

How can my kitty BFF inspire me to have a more *pawsitive* day? (If you get stuck, use your power word.)

_____

pm

3 *pawsitive* things that happened to me today were...

🐾 _____

🐾 _____

🐾 _____

Tonight as I drift off to sleep I will send happiness & *pawsitive* thoughts to...

_____

A cat does not want all the world to love her. Only those she has chosen to love.

HELEN THOMSON

Date _____

My *Pawsitive* Power Word of the Day _____

am

This morning I woke up feeling _____

As I go through my day I wish to feel _____

I am grateful to my cat, _____ because _____

How can my kitty BFF inspire me to have a more *pawsitive* day? (If you get stuck, use your power word.)

pm

3 *pawsitive* things that happened to me today were...

🐾 _____

🐾 _____

🐾 _____

Tonight as I drift off to sleep I will send happiness & *pawsitive* thoughts to...

The difference between ordinary and extraordinary is that little extra.

JIMMY JOHNSON

Date _____

My *Pawsitive* Power Word of the Day _____

am

This morning I woke up feeling _____

As I go through my day I wish to feel _____

I am grateful to my cat, _____ because _____

How can my kitty BFF inspire me to have a more *pawsitive* day? (If you get stuck, use your power word.)

_____

pm

3 *pawsitive* things that happened to me today were...

🐾 _____

🐾 _____

🐾 _____

Tonight as I drift off to sleep I will send happiness & *pawsitive* thoughts to...

_____

If I had a dollar for every time my cat made me smile,
I would be the world's richest person by now.

ERNEST HEMINGWAY

Date _____

My *Pawsitive* Power Word of the Day _____

am

This morning I woke up feeling _____

As I go through my day I wish to feel _____

I am grateful to my cat, _____ because _____

How can my kitty BFF inspire me to have a more *pawsitive* day? (If you get stuck, use your power word.)

pm

3 *pawsitive* things that happened to me today were...

🐾 _____

🐾 _____

🐾 _____

Tonight as I drift off to sleep I will send happiness & *pawsitive* thoughts to...

I discovered that joy is not the negation of pain, but rather acknowledging the presence of pain and feeling happiness in spite of it.

LUPITA NYONG'O

Date _____

My *Pawsitive* Power Word of the Day _____

am

This morning I woke up feeling _____

As I go through my day I wish to feel _____

I am grateful to my cat, _____ because _____

How can my kitty BFF inspire me to have a more *pawsitive* day? (If you get stuck, use your power word.)

pm

3 *pawsitive* things that happened to me today were...

🐾 _____

🐾 _____

🐾 _____

Tonight as I drift off to sleep I will send happiness & *pawsitive* thoughts to...

You didn't save a cat. A cat saved you.

KENDARE BLAKE

Date _____

My *Pawsitive* Power Word of the Day _____

am

This morning I woke up feeling _____

As I go through my day I wish to feel _____

I am grateful to my cat, _____ because _____

How can my kitty BFF inspire me to have a more *pawsitive* day? (If you get stuck, use your power word.)

pm

3 *pawsitive* things that happened to me today were...

🐾 _____

🐾 _____

🐾 _____

Tonight as I drift off to sleep I will send happiness & *pawsitive* thoughts to...

The Pawsitive Monthly Milestone

Make New Friends!

Friends are important for our health, happiness, and longevity. So why not find other cat lovers to connect with? Join a cat lovers' book club, volunteer at a cat shelter, visit a cat café or go to Meetup.com to find some new cat lovin' friends in your area.

Take a selfie of you and your new friends and place it below.

#PawsForTheGoodStuff 🐾 Spread the *Pawsitivity*!

Share your picture with your online community and use #PawsForTheGoodStuff. Together we can change the world, one *pawsitive* moment at a time.

"

Cats never lie about love.

COLETTE

Note to Self

Woohoo — I have two whole *bonus weeks* of journaling coming up!
Boohoo — I *only* have two weeks of journaling left!

Time to order another copy of Paws for the Good Stuff!

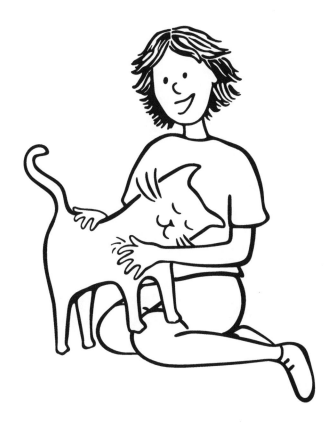

Cats, like butterflies, need no excuse.

ROBERT A. HEINLEIN

Date _____

My *Pawsitive* Power Word of the Day _____

am

This morning I woke up feeling _____

As I go through my day I wish to feel _____

I am grateful to my cat, _____ because _____

How can my kitty BFF inspire me to have a more *pawsitive* day? (If you get stuck, use your power word.)

pm

3 *pawsitive* things that happened to me today were...

🐾 _____

🐾 _____

🐾 _____

Tonight as I drift off to sleep I will send happiness & *pawsitive* thoughts to...

My mission in life is not merely to survive, but to thrive;
and to do so with some passion, some compassion, some humor, and some style.

MAYA ANGELOU

Date _____

My *Pawsitive* Power Word of the Day _____

am

This morning I woke up feeling _____

As I go through my day I wish to feel _____

I am grateful to my cat, _____ because _____

How can my kitty BFF inspire me to have a more *pawsitive* day? (If you get stuck, use your power word.)

_____

pm

3 *pawsitive* things that happened to me today were...

🐾 _____

🐾 _____

🐾 _____

Tonight as I drift off to sleep I will send happiness & *pawsitive* thoughts to...

_____

I cannot imagine not going home to animals.
They are the closest thing to God; they don't harbor resentment.

ELLEN DEGENERES

Date _____

My *Pawsitive* Power Word of the Day _____

am

This morning I woke up feeling _____

As I go through my day I wish to feel _____

I am grateful to my cat, _____ because _____

How can my kitty BFF inspire me to have a more *pawsitive* day? (If you get stuck, use your power word.)

pm

3 *pawsitive* things that happened to me today were...

🐾 _____

🐾 _____

🐾 _____

Tonight as I drift off to sleep I will send happiness & *pawsitive* thoughts to...

Love is the master key that opens the gates of happiness.

OLIVER WENDELL HOLMES

Date _____

My *Pawsitive* Power Word of the Day _____

am

This morning I woke up feeling _____

As I go through my day I wish to feel _____

I am grateful to my cat, _____ because _____

How can my kitty BFF inspire me to have a more *pawsitive* day? (If you get stuck, use your power word.)

pm

3 *pawsitive* things that happened to me today were...

🐾 _____

🐾 _____

🐾 _____

Tonight as I drift off to sleep I will send happiness & *pawsitive* thoughts to...

Cats speak only to those who know how to listen.

SIGMUND FREUD

Date _____

My *Pawsitive* Power Word of the Day _____

am

This morning I woke up feeling _____

As I go through my day I wish to feel _____

I am grateful to my cat, _____ because _____

How can my kitty BFF inspire me to have a more *pawsitive* day? (If you get stuck, use your power word.)

_____

pm

3 *pawsitive* things that happened to me today were...

🐾 _____

🐾 _____

🐾 _____

Tonight as I drift off to sleep I will send happiness & *pawsitive* thoughts to...

_____

There is no stress in the world, only people thinking
stressful thoughts and then acting on them.

DR. WAYNE DYER

Date _____

My *Pawsitive* Power Word of the Day _____

am

This morning I woke up feeling _____

As I go through my day I wish to feel _____

I am grateful to my cat, _____ because _____

How can my kitty BFF inspire me to have a more *pawsitive* day? (If you get stuck, use your power word.)

_____

pm

3 *pawsitive* things that happened to me today were...

🐾 _____

🐾 _____

🐾 _____

Tonight as I drift off to sleep I will send happiness & *pawsitive* thoughts to...

_____

Of all the things God created, from sunrises and rainbows,
to black holes and humor, cats are the most fascinating to me.

JAROD KINTZ

The Seventh Day Challenge

Cats give their hearts to those they love.
What can you give to someone else to brighten their day?
List 5 things below.

1

2

3

4

5

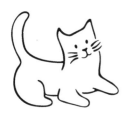

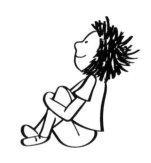

Never confuse a single defeat with a final defeat.

F. SCOTT FITZGERALD

Date _____

My *Pawsitive* Power Word of the Day _____

am

This morning I woke up feeling _____

As I go through my day I wish to feel _____

I am grateful to my cat, _____ because _____

How can my kitty BFF inspire me to have a more *pawsitive* day? (If you get stuck, use your power word.)

pm

3 *pawsitive* things that happened to me today were...

🐾 _____

🐾 _____

🐾 _____

Tonight as I drift off to sleep I will send happiness & *pawsitive* thoughts to...

Cats leave paw prints in your heart, forever and always.

AUTHOR UNKNOWN

Date _____

My *Pawsitive* Power Word of the Day _____

am

This morning I woke up feeling _____

As I go through my day I wish to feel _____

I am grateful to my cat, _____ because _____

How can my kitty BFF inspire me to have a more *pawsitive* day? (If you get stuck, use your power word.)

_____

pm

3 *pawsitive* things that happened to me today were...

🐾 _____

🐾 _____

🐾 _____

Tonight as I drift off to sleep I will send happiness & *pawsitive* thoughts to...

_____

If you're feeling low, don't despair. The sun has a sinking spell every night,
but it comes back up every morning.

DOLLY PARTON

Date _____

My *Pawsitive* Power Word of the Day _____

am

This morning I woke up feeling _____

As I go through my day I wish to feel _____

I am grateful to my cat, _____ because _____

How can my kitty BFF inspire me to have a more *pawsitive* day? (If you get stuck, use your power word.)

_____

pm

3 *pawsitive* things that happened to me today were...

🐾 _____

🐾 _____

🐾 _____

Tonight as I drift off to sleep I will send happiness & *pawsitive* thoughts to...

_____

Cats are the small rays of light who brighten our days for a short time.

CONNIE WILLIS

Date _____

My *Pawsitive* Power Word of the Day _____

am

This morning I woke up feeling _____

As I go through my day I wish to feel _____

I am grateful to my cat, _____ because _____

How can my kitty BFF inspire me to have a more *pawsitive* day? (If you get stuck, use your power word.)

pm

3 *pawsitive* things that happened to me today were...

🐾 _____

🐾 _____

🐾 _____

Tonight as I drift off to sleep I will send happiness & *pawsitive* thoughts to...

The best way out is always through.

ROBERT FROST

Date _____

My *Pawsitive* Power Word of the Day _____

am

This morning I woke up feeling _____

As I go through my day I wish to feel _____

I am grateful to my cat, _____ because _____

How can my kitty BFF inspire me to have a more *pawsitive* day? (If you get stuck, use your power word.)

_____

pm

3 *pawsitive* things that happened to me today were...

🐾 _____

🐾 _____

🐾 _____

Tonight as I drift off to sleep I will send happiness & *pawsitive* thoughts to...

_____

Thou art the Great Cat, the avenger of the Gods, and the judge of words, and the president of the sovereign chiefs and the governor of the holy Circle; thou art indeed... the Great Cat.

INSCRIPTION ON THE ROYAL TOMBS AT THEBES

Date _____

My *Pawsitive* Power Word of the Day _____

am

This morning I woke up feeling _____

As I go through my day I wish to feel _____

I am grateful to my cat, _____ because _____

How can my kitty BFF inspire me to have a more *pawsitive* day? (If you get stuck, use your power word.)

pm

3 *pawsitive* things that happened to me today were...

- 🐾 _____
- 🐾 _____
- 🐾 _____

Tonight as I drift off to sleep I will send happiness & *pawsitive* thoughts to...

Don't cry because it's over, smile because it happened.
DR. SEUSS

The Seventh Day Challenge

Write a gratitude letter to your cat.
Express your appreciation, tenderness, love, and anything else you would like to say.
Don't think about what you are writing, just open your heart, and let the words flow.

The Pawsitive Monthly Milestone

Being Instead of Doing!

Take a break from your busy day to gaze out the window with your cat by your side. Watch the sunset, listen to the birds, feel the joy of having a friend who understands you in a way no one else quite does. Send your BFF your love and gratitude.

Take a few moments to write about your experience.

My Pawsitive Notes

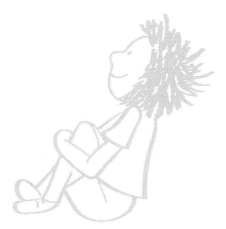

My Pawsitive Notes

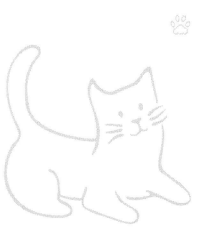

My Pawsitive Notes

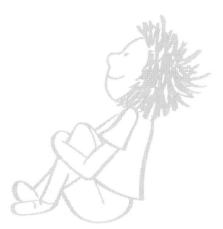

My Pawsitive Notes

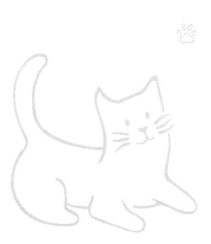

My Pawsitive Notes

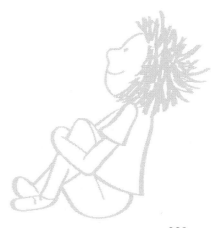

My Pawsitive Notes

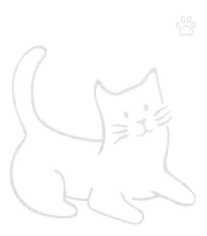

My Pawsitive Notes

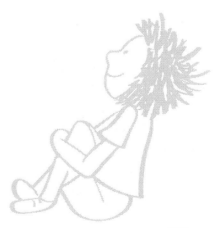

My Pawsitive Notes

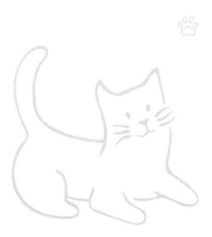

My Pawsitive Notes

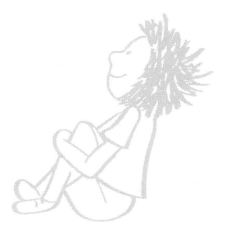

My Pawsitive Notes

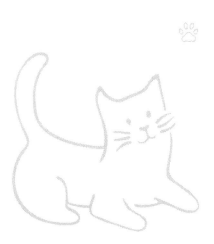

Author Musings

I dearly hope *Paws for the Good Stuff* has enriched your life, shown you what is possible, and created a stronger bond between you and your cat.

Animals do so much for their human friends but it can't all be one - sided; we need to help our animal friends too. And not just the ones in our home but chickens, cows, bears, gorillas, and all sentient creatures we share our magnificent planet with. We are their voice, we are their hope, and together we can make a difference. So please...

🐾 **Adopt don't shop**   🐾 **Be a guardian, not an owner**   🐾 **Go vegan**

If you love animals as much as I do and want the best for them, then we are members of the same tribe. Let's connect!

Join me at *PawsForTheGoodStuff.com* to receive inspiring and *pawsitive* blog posts (I think you will really like them), helpful tips (who doesn't want to make their life better?) and be the first to find out about my upcoming book releases (there's a lot more fun to come).

May your life's journey continue to be enhanced, empowered, and inspired by your fabulous relationships with your animal friends.

Stay *Pawsitive,*

CmDO

P.S. If you enjoyed *Paws for the Good Stuff*, I would really appreciate it if you could take a few moments to leave a short review on Amazon.com or Goodreads.com so other cat lovers can enjoy and learn about it too!

About the Author

Even as a kid, Carlyn Montes De Oca realized that animals have a lot to teach humans about being more human.

Besides being a best-selling award-winning author, Carlyn is also an acupuncturist, keynote speaker, wellness coach, plant-based nutritional consultant, and animal advocate. Her mission is to have the greatest *pawsitive* effect on the lives of animals and the humans who love them.

Carlyn holds a bachelor's degree from Loyola Marymount University in communication arts, a master's degree in Traditional Chinese Medicine from Emperor's College and is certified in plant-based nutrition from the T. Colin Campbell Center for Nutritional Studies at Cornell University.

Carlyn has been featured on television, radio, and dozens of media including ABC, CBS, Fox TV, AARP, and The San Francisco Chronicle.

Voted PETA's Sexiest Vegetarian Over 50, Carlyn has been a spokesperson for the Guardian Campaign at In Defense of Animals and is currently an animal ambassador at Animal Protection of New Mexico.

Carlyn offers workshops, webinars, and wellness coaching. As the founder of The Animal-Human Health Connection, she speaks at animal shelters, non-profits, schools, and corporations on the powerful ways we can improve health, happiness, and longevity through our connection to our animal companions.

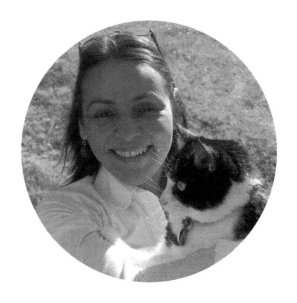

A California native, Carlyn now lives in Santa Fe, New Mexico with her husband Ken Fischer, an award-winning sound editor, and her beloved rescue animals.

Photo by Ken Fischer

Connect with Carlyn

Website AnimalHumanHealth.com
Email cmdo@AnimalHumanHealth.com
Facebook Carlyn Montes De Oca
Twitter CarlynMDO
Instagram Carlyn MontesDeOca
Youtube Carlyn555
Pinterest carlynmdo

An excerpt from

Dog as My Doctor, Cat as My Nurse

Chapter 4

...We can't solve all of our problems by drinking in the exquisite colors of a sunset or feeling an ocean breeze on our face, but these fleeting moments can nurture us in ways that nothing else can. Just ask Michelle, whose cat brings her closer to nature, comforts her, and has given her hope at a time when she has needed it the most.

Abbey, Alley, Mike & Michelle

When we first got married, my husband and I used to take long walks together along the beach in Carpinteria, a small coastal town in southern California. Mike and I loved our time together outdoors, and being so close to nature made us feel lucky.

Mike has Parkinson's disease, and when the disease took a turn for theworse, our lives changed forever. Although Mike pushed bravely forward and tried to maintain his daily activities, he grew more and more physically unstable. Eventually, we came to the realization that we could no longer go out on walks together. This was heartbreaking for both of us.

We moved from the sunny beaches of southern California to Sonoma, four hundred miles north, so Mike could be closer to his family. My daily walks continued, but as I headed out my front door, I felt sad leaving Mike behind.

Excerpt from Dog as My Doctor, Cat as My Nurse *continued...*

One day, I had walked about half a block when out of nowhere I heard a cat chattering up a storm. I turned to find Abbey—our sweet calico cat—trailing along behind me.

We had adopted Abbey from the Humane Society as a kitten. The moment Mike laid eyes on her, he fell in love. There was an indescribable bond between them. We took Abbey home that day, and then, two days later, we went back and got Abbey's sister, Alley.

It had been two years since Mike had stopped walking with me, and now here was Abbey, racing to catch up to me. At first I worried about her darting in front of a car or chasing a lizard, but Abbey stayed right by my side for the entire walk. The next day, she followed me again, and the next day yet again. She has now been my walking partner on this special morning ritual for the last three years. Together we walk under the ornamental pear trees that turn white in the spring. When the winds blow, it looks like you are walking through falling snow. Abbey loves to play with the white leaves as they float to the ground. It's a beautiful sight.

One of the hardest things in the world is to watch helplessly as someone you love suffers from an incurable disease. Mike was once an excellent tennis player and had dreams of traveling the world, but at forty-nine he had to give up those dreams. Somehow, both Abbey and Alley seem to know what Mike needs and when he needs it. At times they snuggle against his legs, purring and kneading him and their touch comforts him. But at other times, when his body becomes rigid, Mike says it feels like his legs are made of cement, and he can't tolerate touch. At these times the cats give Mike his space. They also seem to know when to provide a much-needed laugh, and that's when they will leap into the air or do something funny...

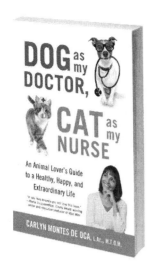

Find out how Michelle and Abbey's story ends — and begins. Pick up your copy of my award-winning book Dog as My Doctor, Cat as My Nurse: An animal lover's guide to a healthy, happy & extraordinary life.

"The Tao of Pooh meets *The Dog Whisperer.*
A must read."

— Readers Favorite Book Review

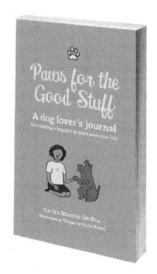

Are you more of a dog lover?
If so, keep an eye out for *Paws the for the Good Stuff: A dog lover's journal for creating a happier & more pawsitive life.*

Get your pawsitive messages, notifications about giveaways, and a heads-up on my upcoming book, *Junkyard Dog: a rescue story,* **at <u>AnimalHumanHealth.com</u>**

Made in the USA
Coppell, TX
27 October 2020

40297341R00134